Cognitive behavioural therapy with schizophrenia

13

Cognitive behavioural therapy with schizophrenia

A PRACTICE MANUAL

By

Hazel E. Nelson

Specialist Services Unit, Horton Hospital, Epsom, UK

Stanley Thornes (Publishers) Ltd

First published 1997 by:
Stanley Thornes (Publishers) Ltd
Ellenborough House
Wellington Street
CHELTENHAM
GL50 1YW
United Kingdom

97 98 99 00 01 / 10 9 8 7 6 5 4 3 2 1

A catalogue record for this book is available from the British Library

ISBN 0-7487-3305-1

Typeset by Acorn Bookwork, Salisbury, Wilts.
Printed and bound in Great Britain by TJ International, Padstow, Cornwall.

Contents

Section 6: LONG-TERM STRATEGIES

Preface

This book is intended for mental health workers who have read about the development and advances that have been made in the use of cognitive behavioural therapy (CBT) with schizophrenia and who want to know how to put these beneficial strategies into practice, effectively and safely. It aims to provide the reader with a range of strategies and techniques, set within a structured framework for the planning and delivery of therapy. It is intended for use as an instruction manual and also as a practice manual to which the therapist can refer when working with individual patients. Formal training in cognitive behavioural therapy with other disorders will no doubt enable the reader to move more quickly through the early sections of this book, but it is not an essential prerequisite for its use. However, it does assume a good working knowledge of schizophrenia and practical experience with the many different and diverse ways that this disorder can affect people and is directed at clinically qualified staff working in this area.

This is a practical guide, not an academic textbook, and as such it does not include descriptions or discussions of the extensive research literatures, which have been comprehensively covered elsewhere (see pp. 244–5). It should be noted that as this book concentrates on those aspects of CBT that are relevant to and have been developed specifically for use with schizophrenia, it will not provide the reader with the knowledge or the practical techniques necessary to work with other disorders to which CBT is often applied, such as depression and anxiety.

The principal aim of cognitive behavioural therapy with people with schizophrenia is to relieve their distress, to improve their sense of well-being and the quality of their lives. When used as a treatment for delusions and hallucinations, CBT aims to reduce the distress that these symptoms can cause and to provide the person with strategies and skills to manage residual symptoms in everyday life. The primary aim is not a reduction in the symptoms *per se*, though this usually follows as a result of successful treatment.

The first section of the treatment manual describes the basic principles underpinning the cognitive behavioural model and how they relate to the development, maintenance and modification of delusions and hallucinations. The second section considers what it might be like to experience these symptoms and recommends ways of improving the therapeutic alliance and overcoming problems that may occur during therapy. Section 3 discusses the ethical issues around treating people for an illness that they may deny having and shows why it is essential, when setting the goals for therapy, to take into account the possible impact on the patient of removing or modifying his delusions or hallucinations. Having taken the reader from the initial meeting with the patient through the assessment and planning stages, Sections 4 and 5 detail the different strategies that can be used with delusions and hallucinations, respectively. Section 6 deals with long-term strategies.

The CBT strategies described in this book are those that we have found to be the most useful in our work with the patients in our Specialist Services Unit, a unit for people with medication-resistant and enduring schizophrenia. The people referred to our unit are those who have failed to respond adequately to the treatments available in the admissions wards, so they are amongst the most severely affected by their illness. Nevertheless, we have found that there are few people for whom we can do absolutely nothing and even small gains in this seriously ill and disadvantaged group must be considered worthwhile. The strategies are equally if not more effective with less severely ill people and progress is usually faster.

All the clinical examples and cases described in this book are based on people with whom we have worked over the past ten years, but inessential details have been changed in order to protect the identities of the individuals concerned.

Note on terminology

When referring to someone with schizophrenia I have used the term 'patient' rather than 'client' because I believe it is a perfectly respectable term to use, not least because we are all patients at some time in our lives. As we shall see later in this book, we can inadvertently imply things by the words we use and I think this is a case in point. By using the term 'client' I think we risk subtly implying to the people we work with that we are not referring to them as patients because being a patient is somehow 'not nice' – which, I am sure, is the exact opposite of what people who studiously avoid using the term 'patient' actually intend to imply. In clinical practice I would normally refer to someone with schizophrenia as 'someone with schizophrenia' rather than 'a patient', but unfortunately this phrase is too cumbersome to use repeatedly in a written text.

When I am writing of a patient or a therapist in general, I have used the terms 'he', 'his' and 'him' rather than the clumsy 's/he', 'his/her' and 'him/her' or the grammatically incorrect 'they', 'their' and 'them'. I appreciate that this may verge on what is currently considered to be 'politically incorrect' use of language, and if this is so then I must beg the reader's indulgence, but it does make the text easier to read and that was my primary concern.

Acknowledgements

It has been a very real privilege and pleasure to know and work with the patients at Horton Hospital over the past ten years; the best in the book is what they have given me. I have been fortunate in the generous co-operation and interest shown to me by my colleagues in the two multidisciplinary teams in which I work; in particular, I would like to express my gratitude to Professor Tom Barnes and to Dr John Robertson for all their much appreciated support over the years. I have been fortunate, also, to be part of a stimulating District Psychology Department; my thanks go particularly to Lesley Parkinson for her infectious enthusiasm and assistance.

I am indebted to Janet Grimshaw and Sue Benthall for their unfailing efficiency, patience and good humour in the preparation of this manuscript; my warmest thanks go to them both. I am grateful to Hamish McLeod and Penny Strover for taking the time to read the penultimate draft and for their helpful comments on it.

A special thank you goes to my daughter, Hilary, for all the encouragement and help that she has given me during this project.

The cognitive behavioural approach to therapy

1

INTRODUCTION

Most people who seek psychological therapy do so because of the unpleasant way they feel. The principal aim of cognitive therapy in these cases is to alleviate the unpleasant feelings, but cognitive therapy does not tackle these feelings directly; rather, it seeks to achieve the required changes by modifying the thoughts (hence the term 'cognitive' therapy) and beliefs that underlie them.

CORE CONCEPTS OF THE COGNITIVE BEHAVIOURAL MODEL

The relationship between thoughts, feelings and beliefs

A central concept for the cognitive behavioural model of therapy is the relationship that exists between our thoughts and our feelings. This states that the way we feel about a situation or experience depends on what we think about it and how we interpret it. For example, two people are given surprise birthday presents of a balloon ride. One thinks 'That will be exciting, how kind of my partner to go to such trouble and expense', leading to feelings of pleasurable anticipation and affection, whereas the other thinks 'I will feel frightened the whole trip, what a waste of money', leading to feelings of fear and annoyance.

Another core concept for cognitive therapy is that the thoughts we have about a situation, the way we interpret it, are influenced by our beliefs about ourselves and the world. In the example just given, the first person believed that ballooning is exciting rather than dangerous and that his partner cared enough for him to try to give him a present he would really like. In contrast, the second person believed that ballooning is dangerous and that his partner was uncaring about what would please him.

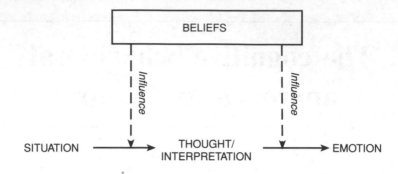

Fig. 1.1   The relationship between thoughts, feelings and beliefs.

In the above example, the same situation led to different thoughts and hence to different feelings, but it is also true that the same thought can lead to different emotional responses in different people. For example, a child and an elderly person may both think on looking out and seeing a snowfall 'It's slippery out there, I will slide and fall over', but the emotional responses to this thought will be quite different. The child, believing that sliding is fun and that falling over will cause him only minor discomfort, will be unconcerned or even excited by the thought of sliding on the snow, whereas the elderly person, believing that he could be seriously hurt, will be fearful at the same thought. Once again, it is the beliefs that the person brings to a situation that influence the basic **situation→thought→emotion** process, this time by influencing the emotions that are produced by the thought.

The symptom maintenance cycle

We have looked at the way in which our thoughts affect our feelings and emotions, but our thoughts can have other effects as well. In the CBT literature these effects are generally termed 'symptoms' because any one of them can be the symptom that causes the patient to seek therapy.

Our thoughts and interpretations of situations have an effect on our behaviour and our motivation to act. In the example given previously of the balloon ride, the recipient who interpreted the gift as a sign of his partner's caring thoughtfulness is likely to respond in a warm, affectionate way whereas the recipient who interpreted it in the opposite way is likely to respond in a cold, hurt or angry manner.

Our thoughts can also affect our physiology: these responses are particularly important for anxiety-based disorders and can be amongst the most unpleasant symptoms of these disorders. They can affect behaviour directly or lead to other fearful thoughts, for example the agoraphobic

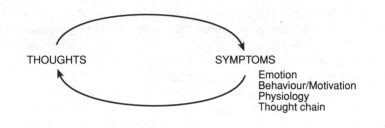

Fig. 1.2 The symptom maintenance cycle.

who interprets his racing heart as a sign of an impending heart attack. In schizophrenia, physiological responses of anxiety may be given a delusional explanation which then exacerbates the anxiety; for example, one of our patients was frightened that he was being invaded by aliens and interpreted the unpleasant sensations in his body as confirmation that they were getting into him.

Thoughts flow through our minds in a steady stream, so it is not surprising to find that thoughts can also produce other thoughts that lead to other thoughts and so on. This has been called the **thought chain**. For example, an A-level student waking up in the early hours on the morning of his exam might think 'It's only 3am – I've only had four hours sleep – if I can't get back to sleep I will be tired in the morning – if I'm tired I won't do well in the exam – if I don't do well in the exam I won't get my university place – if I don't get my university place I will be unemployed and have to stay at home – I'll be a failure, my life will be ruined'. The importance of these thought chains is that each and any one of the thoughts in the chain can produce its own set of 'symptoms'. In the example just given, it is not the thought that it is 3am that is producing the strong emotions of panic and dread or even the thought that the exam is only seven hours away, but rather the thoughts further down the chain about his life being in ruins if he is unable to take up his university place.

The effects that thoughts have on emotions and the other so-called symptoms would not, by themselves, be such a problem if they just faded away after being triggered. The problem is that these 'symptoms' tend to influence subsequent thoughts in such a way as to maintain or exacerbate the existing emotional state. Note how this effect works for all the examples given above. The thoughts/symptoms relationship is therefore a two-way one as the thoughts produce the symptoms but then the symptoms influence the thoughts: this is often called the **symptom mainte-**

nance cycle because it tends to act so as to keep the mood and thoughts from changing. (It should be noted that although the symptom maintenance cycle is generally talked about in CBT writings with regard to the maintenance of negative thoughts and emotions, the same process also works to maintain positive thoughts and emotions. This means that if during therapy you are able to modify the thoughts and emotions so that they become positive rather than negative, then the thoughts/symptoms cycle will work in the patient's favour to maintain this positive state of affairs.)

Automatic thoughts

The term **automatic thought** occurs frequently in writings about cognitive behavioural therapy, often as part of the term **negative automatic thought** (NAT). Automatic thoughts can be positive, neutral or negative in their effects on a person, but since psychotherapy is primarily concerned with those thoughts that have the negative, unwanted effects, negative automatic thoughts are the ones most commonly talked about in connection with CBT. (Note: When used in CBT, the terms **negative** and **positive** refer only to the effect the thought has on the person concerned; they do not imply any moral or other value.)

Our brains are generating thoughts all the time that we are awake. These thoughts can be about any aspect of the situation that we are in, including what it means, how it might develop and how we might respond to those developments, or they can be about other things quite unrelated to the present situation. This constant stream of thoughts is necessary for our survival and often acts as the trigger for our more purposeful thinking. Automatic thoughts are constantly monitored by the part of our brain responsible for the overall executive control of our thoughts and actions (found in the front part of the brain, behind our foreheads); this central executive part of the brain selects the most relevant automatic thoughts for further attention, at which stage we become aware of them as conscious thoughts. Unlike purposeful thinking, when you follow a deliberate train of thought within conscious awareness (e.g. in working out the solution to a problem), automatic thoughts are not under our conscious control but occur spontaneously and effortlessly, much as dreams occur spontaneously and without conscious control during sleep.

Characteristics of automatic thoughts

1. Automatic thoughts occur spontaneously and without effort from the person concerned. They cannot be switched off or consciously controlled.

2. Though often verbal (i.e. occurring as words), automatic thoughts can also occur as images or in a vague, preverbal form. They often occur as fragments or partial thoughts, flashing rapidly through the brain.
3. Automatic thoughts may be sensible but they can also be unreasonable, impossible or even bizarre.
4. If automatic thoughts do not come to conscious awareness their content cannot be recognised or subjected to rational thinking, but nevertheless they may still evoke a strong, emotional reaction.
5. Automatic thoughts may reflect the thinker's underlying belief system about himself and the world, but not necessarily so. One can have an automatic thought about anything within one's memory or knowledge system, i.e. about anything one has ever seen, heard, read or imagined.

The role that automatic thoughts may play in producing an emotional response or mood state is a key feature of the cognitive behavioural therapy model, especially as the latter was originally developed for work with depression. It was recognised that a depressed feeling or mood could be triggered by a thought flashing through the subject's mind, even though the subject was not consciously aware of the thought. CBT with people with schizophrenia tends to concentrate more on the thoughts and beliefs that are in the patient's conscious awareness, but nevertheless you should be aware of the possibility that automatic thoughts, of which the person is not consciously aware, could be relevant: you should be particularly sensitive to this latter possibility where the emotional response does not appear to be consistent with the thoughts and beliefs reported by the patient.

Beliefs and belief systems

(Note: The term **belief system** is used rather loosely in CBT literature. It means a cohesive collection of beliefs but may be used to refer to a subset of beliefs around a particular topic, e.g. religious beliefs, or to the sum total set of beliefs held by that person.)

The function of beliefs

We all have a unique set of beliefs which represent our particular way of generalising about the world and our part in it. Without beliefs we would be unable to cope with the complexity and variability of our lives. Because we are social animals it is essential that we are able to manoeuvre our way through the ever-changing social situations around us and so it is not surprising that many of our beliefs concern ourselves, others and interactions between ourselves and others.

Beliefs are our 'best bet' estimates of how things operate in the world, which enable us to understand what is going on and to respond appropriately without having to treat each and every situation as if it were new. For example, I have developed the belief that someone smiling and approaching me with an outstretched hand is a sign of friendly non-aggression and so I am able to respond appropriately to this situation whenever it occurs; but if I had no belief about this behaviour I would have to consider all the possible reasons for the outstretched hand, smile and movement towards me and weigh these up before being able to work out a suitable response. It is easy to see that we would simply be overwhelmed if we did not have beliefs to short-cut the lengthy process of rationally analysing every situation we encountered. Because we have developed beliefs to cover most situations we only have to resort to analysing a situation more rationally (a) on the very rare occasions when the situation is so novel that no relevant belief has been developed or (b) when it is not clear which of two or more beliefs is the appropriate one; for example, if somebody approaches me smiling but with raised hand as if to strike, then I have to decide whether my belief about smiling indicating non-aggression or my belief about upraised hands indicating threat is the more appropriate one in that situation. Even in situations where there is more than one belief that is relevant to the situation, the existence of those beliefs greatly reduces the range of possibilities that have to be weighed up and thought through rationally. Note that in some cases even incorrect or dysfunctional beliefs may be better than having no beliefs at all because they allow a response to be made quickly, even though it may not be the best possible response for the person concerned.

Functional and dysfunctional beliefs
Beliefs may be described as functional or dysfunctional. Functional beliefs are those that are useful to the person, that serve a positive function; for example, the belief 'If I put my hand in a fire, it will hurt' protects my hand from physical damage, whilst the belief 'Everyone makes mistakes sometimes, even really successful people' protects me from feeling a failure when I make errors. Dysfunctional beliefs are those that are unhelpful to the person holding them, that have an overall negative effect; for example, the belief 'I am an even better driver when I'm drunk' increases the risk of self-injury and a drink-driving charge whilst the belief 'It's a sign of weakness to cry' means that on some occasions I may not only feel very sad but also ashamed for showing those feelings. (Note: As with the terms **positive** and **negative**, the terms **functional** and **dysfunctional** do not imply a moral assessment about the belief but are a purely practical description of how beneficial or harmful the belief is for that person.)

Not all beliefs are **either** functional **or** dysfunctional.

1. A belief may be functional in some contexts but dysfunctional in others. For example, the belief 'It's OK to retaliate with physical force if attacked' may be functional if you are trapped in an alleyway by someone threatening a violent assault but it would be dysfunctional for someone working in a mental health setting.
2. Similarly, a belief that is functional at some time in the person's life may become dysfunctional or vice versa. For example, the belief 'I should put myself first' might be functional for a young person striving to achieve independence and career success but would be highly dysfunctional as a parent.
3. Within a single context, the belief may be both functional and dysfunctional at the same time, that is, it may be functional in some ways and dysfunctional in others. For example, the belief 'It's dangerous to go out after dark' is functional in that it avoids the risk of getting attacked but is dysfunctional in that it limits social activity.

Beliefs that would be appropriate and functional for most occasions may be dysfunctional if they are held in an extreme or rigid way that does not allow for human frailty or the exceptional circumstances that can occur in life, e.g. the belief 'I should always be kind to my fellow men' or 'It's wrong to behave aggressively'. Beliefs of this kind are often expressed in terms of 'always', 'never', 'every', 'none', etc., and often include the word 'should'. In contrast, functional beliefs tend to be expressed in less extreme forms and to allow exceptions to the general rule, for example, 'It's wrong to kill (except as a soldier in wartime)'.

By their very nature, functional beliefs tend to benefit the person holding them and it is a sign of a normal, healthy psychological state that we tend to believe things that go in our favour and to ignore or reject things that go against us. Thus, we tend to have a rosier view of ourselves and of other people's opinions of us than is actually true in fact, the so-called **self-serving bias**. We are also biased in that we tend to adopt beliefs that have the potential to show us in a good light. For example, you may have noticed amongst your friends and acquaintances that people who are good at sport tend to value sporting prowess as an important achievement whereas people who play musical instruments consider musical ability a more important characteristic.

The organisation of beliefs

Although we have no direct evidence of where or how beliefs are organised and stored in the brain, their apparent resistance to the effects of focal and generalised brain damage strongly suggests that they must be stored in some diffuse way. We know that our knowledge system is organised into interconnecting networks and subsystems and it may well be that our belief systems are similarly organised. This would be compatible with the way that new beliefs tend to be adapted to fit into the existing belief system.

The key function of a belief system is to bring cohesion and order to the world, to enable us to make predictions and to act accordingly, so it is important that our beliefs do not result in conflicting interpretations or predictions. Therefore, although some inconsistencies can be tolerated within a belief system, for the most part directly opposing or conflicting beliefs are not tolerated. Contradictory beliefs can coexist if undetected, but once a situation occurs that calls them into conflict then it is usual for either or both the beliefs to be modified to return harmony to the system. Modification may require one belief to be discarded but is more often achieved by adding provisos to one or more of the beliefs. For example, if you were to hold the beliefs 'It's wrong to tell lies' and 'It's wrong to hurt people's feelings' then these would be called into direct conflict if a friend asked you how you liked her new (unattractive) hairstyle, since you would have to act against one of your beliefs. In practice, you are likely to resolve the conflict either by modifying your belief about telling lies ('It's generally wrong to tell lies but it's permissible to save someone's feelings'), which would allow you to answer 'Yes, it looks good' or by modifying your belief about hurting people ('Sometimes it's necessary to hurt people's feelings to be kind in the long run'), which would allow you to answer 'Your old style looked better'. Note that failure to modify one of the beliefs would necessarily result in your feeling guilty, either for telling lies or for hurting someone's feelings.

Situations in everyday life are complex so that more than one belief or belief system may be activated. Despite developing belief systems that are, on the whole, internally consistent, these activated beliefs may lead to contradictory interpretations of events or to opposing actions. For example, a mother taking a child for inoculation may bring to the situation a belief that she should protect her child against illnesses and a belief that she should not cause her child pain. In such cases the potential conflict is resolved by one belief taking precedence over the other. Which belief takes precedence will depend not only on the relative strength of the beliefs but also on the circumstances and the possible outcomes. Thus, in the above case, the mother might decide to proceed with even a very painful inoculation if the illness was severe, whereas she might decide against it if the illness was a mild one. Alternatively, if the injection caused only mild pain then she might decide to go ahead with the inoculation even for a mild illness.

Some of our beliefs, especially those about social matters, can be remarkably fluid. For example, on some occasions I may feel full of self-confidence but on other occasions I may have a much poorer opinion of myself. Similarly, most of us do not have stable beliefs about our attractiveness, work competence, popularity, etc. Fluctuations in our beliefs can be affected by external factors, for example where we are and whom we are with, and also by internal factors. A very important internal factor affecting beliefs about ourselves and others is our mood; for example, if I feel happy I am more likely to believe that I am attractive to other people, competent at work, etc. than if I feel depressed.

Belief formation

Our beliefs develop from our experience of the world, using the term experience in its widest sense. This includes internally generated experiences (thoughts, feelings, imagination, etc.) as well as our direct experiences of the world (including childhood experiences). It also includes what we learn about other people's experiences, through education, books, TV, etc. The beliefs we develop are heavily influenced by the cultural (including religious, social and political) beliefs of those around us; the beliefs of personally significant others, such as our family, friends, peer groups, etc., are particularly important. The beliefs we develop are also affected to some extent by our biological predisposition, which can be likened to the hard wiring of a computer and includes both the predispositions that we all share as human beings, for example to protect members of our own family, and those that vary from one person to another, for example, the tendency to be anxious. At a more temporary biological level, mood state may also influence the development of beliefs; for example, a person will more readily develop negative beliefs about himself and the world when he is depressed.

New beliefs are heavily influenced by the existing belief system because the existing beliefs bias the perception and interpretation of new information. In this way, new beliefs tend to develop that are compatible with the existing belief system and will fit in without causing inconsistencies. However, should the new belief contradict and be held more strongly than a pre-existing belief, then the latter has to be changed or adapted in order to incorporate the new belief.

Belief maintenance: The self-confirming belief circles

Biased interpretations (see Fig. 1.3(a))

Situations are interpreted according to our individual beliefs; these interpretations then serve to reinforce our existing beliefs because they are consistent with those beliefs. In this way beliefs are powerful reinforcers of themselves. A clear illustration of this effect from everyday life is that

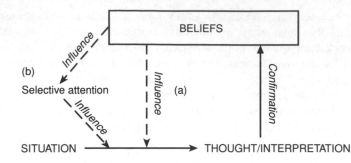

Fig. 1.3 Beliefs confirm themselves by influencing the perception and interpretation of evidence.

of belief in the accuracy of horoscopes. Suppose the New Year's 'Star Predictions' claim that a world leader will be assassinated in the early part of the year. In May, the ruler of a minor country is killed in a military coup and there are no other assassinations of political leaders that year. The reader who believes that horoscopes can predict the future will point to this assassination as the event foretold by the horoscope, an interpretation that the reader will triumphantly assume to provide further evidence to support his already existing belief in the accuracy of horoscopes. Another reader believes that it is impossible to predict the future from the stars and equally triumphantly points out that once again the horoscopes were inaccurate since the only political assassination that year was of the leader of a small country, not a world leader, and that May is not the early part of the year. By this interpretation the second reader's belief in the inaccuracies of horoscopes has also been confirmed. Thus the same event has been interpreted in completely different ways but in both cases in such a way as to reinforce the existing belief.

If a belief is very strongly held, the distortion can be so extreme that even blatantly contradictory evidence is interpreted as supporting the belief; for example, the overconfident job applicant may put his failure to get the post down to the fact that the bosses were worried about employing someone who knew more about the work than they did.

Selective attention (see Fig. 1.3(b))

A second important factor in the maintenance of beliefs is that of selective attention, whereby people tend to notice evidence that confirms their existing beliefs and to ignore or trivialise evidence that is contradictory. For example, people who believe in the ability of spirit mediums to pass on messages from the dead will take notice of the instances when a medium seemed to be uncannily accurate with a name or piece of personal knowledge ('She couldn't possibly have known his name was Harry!') whereas the unbeliever would notice all the mistakes and messages that did not make sense ('No-one knew of anyone who had died recently in a car accident' and 'The message about washing up didn't make sense to anyone').

The self-confirming circles

The effects of selective attention and distorted interpretation are powerful indeed for belief maintenance since the joint operation of these processes ensures that contradictory evidence is either ignored, dismissed or, in extreme cases, interpreted in such a distorted way as to be no longer contradictory. At the same time, attention is given to confirmatory evidence, or neutral evidence that has been interpreted in a confirmatory way, so that the belief is strengthened.

The stronger the belief, the more likely it is that evidence contrary to it will be ignored or distorted. The fact that we distort evidence in this way is not, as one might at first think, a weakness in our psychological system. One of the key functions of a belief is to bring stability to our world and enable us to respond consistently to it. In this variable world in which we live it is advantageous to us to have beliefs that, once formed, can resist the influence of isolated contradictory evidence. If this were not the case our beliefs would be in a constant state of change and stability would be lost. Furthermore, since our beliefs are normally based on experience and evidence accumulated over some time, it is generally appropriate not to change them on the basis of the occasional contradiction. By their very nature, beliefs are generalities about how things are in the world and so exceptions would be expected. Normally, it is only when contradictory evidence becomes overwhelming that we change our beliefs to accommodate it; the more firmly held the belief, the greater the contradictory evidence required to bring about this change.

The self-confirmation of delusional beliefs

Thus we see that it is not just people with delusions who do not treat evidence concerning their beliefs in an objective way; none of us do. Indeed, with respect to the effects of selective attention and distortion of interpretation, delusional beliefs appear to behave in very much the same way as any other strongly held belief. It is only because the delusional beliefs of people with schizophrenia are alien to our own beliefs that we can so readily see the distortions that are going on in the deluded person's thinking. One only has to think of friends or acquaintances who hold different views from oneself to see how 'blind' people can be to contradictory evidence and how they can distort the facts; and how

frustrating it can be that they are apparently quite unaware of their prejudiced thinking! On the other hand, when we are with people who share
our beliefs it will be virtually impossible for us to detect the biases in our
thinking, because they are never exposed as such.

Of course, it is important to realise that although we are confident that
we see things clearly, objectively and without bias, this is not the case.
We cannot avoid bringing our beliefs to every situation that we encounter
or distorting our interpretation of situations according to our own beliefs.
This includes our therapy sessions and this is why it is so important for
us to try to be aware of our own beliefs and prejudices and the influence
they may have on our performance as therapists.

Belief modification

We have already noted that some beliefs, especially those about social
matters, are not fixed; they can vary and fluctuate according to our mood
and circumstances. For example, our self-confidence can vary according
to the situation we are in and according to biological factors such as
alcohol or hormone levels or our mood state. We can even hold apparently opposite beliefs that can be elicited in different circumstances. For
instance, as I sit at my desk writing this paragraph, I hold a firm belief
that ghosts do not exist, but I have a suspicion that if I were left alone at
night, in the dark, in an allegedly haunted house, then the firmness of
this belief would evaporate!

The fact that incompatible beliefs can be triggered in different circumstances (e.g. I am good at my work/I am poor at my work; ghosts do not
exist/ghosts might well exist) has an interesting implication for the theory
of what we are actually doing in cognitive therapy when we say that we
'modify' a belief. If opposing beliefs can be elicited from the same person
in different circumstances, then this suggests that both beliefs must be
held somewhere within the overall belief system and that the belief that is
triggered to operate in any one situation, i.e. the belief that predominates,
will depend on a complex of internal (mental) and external (environ-
mental) factors. It seems likely, therefore, that what happens during
therapy is not that the old belief is irrevocably changed into the new
belief but rather that the new belief is established and strengthened so
that in most circumstances it is this new belief that will be activated
rather than the old one.

The notion that new beliefs **overlie** old ones rather than erasing and
replacing them would account for the apparent fluidity of beliefs which
can be seen in our everyday lives as well as the fluctuations that can
occur with delusional beliefs. For example, the overlaying of beliefs
would account for my irrational fear if I were to be left alone in the
haunted house. I was brought up in a culture where ghost stories were

read and incidents of hauntings were seriously discussed, so at one time I believed that at least there was a possibility that ghosts could exist. Acquisition of an understanding of the laws of physics and a closer scrutiny of the evidence from this viewpoint convinced me that ghosts cannot exist as a physical, visible entity and it is this belief that is activated in all normal circumstances. Nevertheless, the earlier belief about ghosts is still stored somewhere in my nervous system, ready to be reactivated given the right circumstances. Since I have always understood that ghosts tend to haunt specific places, being in a reputedly haunted house at night would be just the sort of external situation most likely to trigger my old belief about ghosts. Even so, this might not be enough on its own to activate the belief but if I was in a state of anxiety, provoked by being on my own in a dark and unknown place, then the external and internal conditions taken together would almost certainly be enough to trigger the old belief. Once the old belief had been triggered then neutral events would be interpreted and distorted in line with that old belief. For example, once I believed ghosts to be possible then the cool draught of air and creaking sound from the stairs would take on a new and a sinister significance . . .

Biases in thinking (errors of thinking)

Our thinking and interpretation of events are influenced not only by the beliefs that we bring to a situation but also by the ways in which we think about things. We all exhibit biases in thinking (what were called 'errors of thinking' in the early CBT literature) from time to time, for example jumping to conclusions on the basis of inadequate evidence; indeed, our thinking is probably mildly distorted for most of the time. Not that we are aware of most of these distortions; they tend to lead to conclusions that are consistent with our existing beliefs and hence are accepted by us without question. As we have already seen, it is generally only those thoughts that contradict our beliefs that are considered more critically.

Biases in thinking are a particularly important factor in depression because when people are in a depressed mood they are particularly likely to be biased in their thinking; for example, so-called black-and-white thinking may lead the patient to conclude he is either a total success or a total failure, with no position possible in between. These biases can be severe, leading to significant distortions in rational thinking, such as categorising oneself as a failure because of one error made at work.

People with schizophrenia do show biases in thinking, especially related to their delusional beliefs, but probably no more so than anyone else with beliefs held with the same degree of conviction. The biases in schizophrenic thinking may be more apparent to those of us with more 'normal' beliefs because the conclusions produced by their distortions are more obviously 'wrong', but most of us are capable of equally prejudiced and distorted thinking when it comes to our strongly held beliefs (e.g. our political or religious beliefs), distortions that go undetected when we are mixing with like-minded people but that are readily criticised by people of dissimilar persuasion. Thus, people with schizophrenia do concentrate on evidence confirming their delusions and pass over evidence that contradicts them but, as we have already seen, this is a feature of normal cognitive processing. Similarly, people with schizophrenia do jump to conclusions on the basis of inadequate evidence, but this also is a tendency that we all suffer from to some degree. The one error of thinking that probably does occur more frequently in schizophrenia than in non-psychotic people is that of 'personalisation' or 'self-reference'. Although we all tend to attribute more significance to ourselves in the grand scheme of things than is objectively justified, people with schizophrenia can be extreme when making this error; in its most extreme form, this bias is what the psychiatric literature calls a delusion of self-reference. However, as far as treatment is concerned, it is not possible to approach delusions of self-reference as one would approach biases of thinking in depression or anxiety-based disorders because, without insight, the patient is unable to use the concept in a therapeutic way; he **knows** his conclusions are correct and therefore he **knows** that his thinking is sound. It would only be possible to work with biases of self-reference in the standard CBT way after the patient had gained insight about the nature of his delusions, by which time treatment would already be well advanced.

Since most patients with schizophrenia do not seem to be abnormally prone to biased thinking, this is not an important area for treatment. Furthermore, in our clinical experience we have found that attempting to work with biases in thinking in the standard CBT way, with thought diaries and homework assignments, is generally not productive. This is partly because our patients are mostly unwilling/unable to do written homework assignments, but also because they find it difficult to work at the abstract level of thinking about thinking. For these reasons, this particular part of the standard CBT model is not described further in this book; readers interested in this aspect of treatment should consult the CBT books on the treatment of depression.

GENERAL MODEL FOR COGNITIVE BEHAVIOURAL THERAPY

Figure 1.4 draws together the different aspects of the cognitive behavioural model described in the earlier parts of this chapter. When applied in clinical practice, this model can be used to describe and define

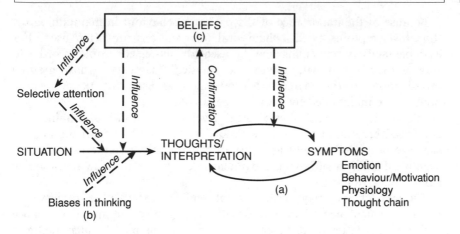

Fig. 1.4 A general model for CBT.

the patient's problem in terms of the psychological processes involved. Accurate assessment and formulation of the problem is a necessary prerequisite for the planning and delivery of the most appropriate line of therapy. This formulation may be updated as therapy progresses and new information comes in, and the treatment plan is adjusted accordingly.

Patients referred for CBT usually come for treatment because of some unpleasant mood state (e.g. depression) or emotional response to situations (e.g. anxiety), or because of the behavioural consequences of the emotional response (e.g. phobia). Treatment does not target the emotional state directly but attempts to modify it indirectly, by modifying the factors that cause or influence it. Using the model for CBT depicted in Figure 1.4 there are three main lines of treatment:

The maintaining thoughts/symptoms cycle (a)

This is especially important for anxiety-based disorders where the powerful physiological responses of anxiety/fear may produce other frightening thoughts (e.g. 'My heart is pounding so fast, I may get a heart attack') that develop their own fear-maintaining cycle and where changes in motivation and behaviour (especially avoidant behaviour) will act so as to protect the fearful thoughts from change. Similarly, depression commonly affects motivation and behaviour (e.g. withdrawal from social contacts and activities) in a way that prevents opportunities for the mood to lift, and depressed mood will produce mood-congruent chains of thought, often distorted by biases in thinking. The CBT intervention can be at any part(s) of the cycle, the aim being to break a negative cycle and to re-establish a more positive one.

Because of the importance of the patient's behaviour in maintaining the thoughts/symptoms cycle, behavioural interventions are often used. For example, activity scheduling may be used for depressed people in order to reverse their social withdrawal and physical inactivity, whilst gradual introduction to the feared situation may be used for people whose phobias are maintained by avoidant behaviours.

Interventions at the physiological level (e.g. relaxation training and controlled breathing) may help with anxiety-based disorders if the unpleasant symptoms of anxiety are part of the thoughts/symptoms cycle, for example if the fear of having a panic attack is preventing the agoraphobic from leaving home.

Thought chains may develop that end in extreme or exaggerated thoughts which themselves may develop thoughts/symptoms maintenance cycles. If this latter occurs then the thought chains may be identified and CBT techniques used to break each of these supporting or exacerbating thoughts/symptoms maintenance cycles.

Biases in thinking (b)

This aspect of CBT treatment is particularly important for depressive disorders because depressed people are particularly prone to making significant distortions in their interpretations of situations and in their thinking. Treatment is aimed at helping the person to recognise when he is making an error of thinking, to identify what distortion this has led to and to challenge the thoughts. In this way he learns to generate more rational and positive interpretations of situations, which in turn leads to improvement in mood state.

The underlying beliefs (c)

If the unwanted symptoms cannot be shifted by the above two approaches then it may be necessary to attempt direct modification of the underlying beliefs. This approach tends to be the last of the three used because beliefs, particularly those that are deeply held or have been held for a long time, may be difficult to identify and modify and so treatment at this level tends to take much longer. However, if belief modification does not occur as a result of treatment at levels (a) or (b), then some more direct belief modification work will be necessary in order to progress the treatment and to avoid relapse after treatment ceases.

Personality disorders are rooted in dysfunctional beliefs at the core schemata level (i.e. fundamental beliefs about the self and the world) and treatment at the belief level in these cases typically takes years to show significant positive effects. Working on the belief system is also the essence of CBT with delusions, but although delusional beliefs may be held very strongly the fact that they developed later in life means that they are potentially less imbedded and enmeshed with other beliefs than dysfunctional schemata and therefore in this respect they are potentially easier to shift.

CBT with accurate and inaccurate interpretations of reality

Much of CBT is concerned with factually inaccurate interpretations of reality, for example the depressed young man who thinks his partner is about to leave him because the partner came home late from work, or the social phobic who fears that everyone will look critically at him when he enters a party. In these circumstances, helping the patient to make more realistic and accurate interpretations of situations will result in more positive thoughts and hence more positive emotions. As a general rule, if an interpretation of an event or situation is factually inaccurate then it is appropriate to work on modifying the inaccuracies of interpretation. However, if the interpretation is factually accurate then it would be inappropriate to attempt to modify the interpretation itself; instead, therapy would attempt to relieve the unpleasant emotions by changing the beliefs surrounding the interpretation. For example, if the young man just mentioned is correct in his interpretation of his partner's behaviour, then his despair about ever being happy again could only be relieved by modifying his belief that he could never be happy with anyone else.

THE THERAPIST IN COGNITIVE BEHAVIOURAL THERAPY

The therapy

Cognitive therapy is a joint venture between the patient and the therapist. Both participants in this venture are of equal status; generally speaking, the patient is the 'expert' about his experiences, thoughts, feelings, beliefs, etc. whilst the therapist is the 'expert' in possible ways of changing these.

Cognitive therapy aims to achieve the patient's goals: the only exception to this would be if the patient's goals would adversely and unfairly affect others. If the initial goals are not realistic or practicable, they are discussed with the patient so that achievable and useful goals can be set. (But see Chapter 3 for some of the problems in discussing goals for delusional beliefs with the patient.)

The therapeutic process

One of the basic principles of the CBT method of working is that the therapist does not tell the patient or give information directly but rather guides the patient's thinking along the right tracks (and hopefully to the right conclusions) by asking appropriate questions. This is known as the method of **Socratic dialogue** or **questioning**, so called after its use in texts written over 2000 years ago by Plato in which he would develop his philosophical argument by reporting a dialogue between Socrates and a philosophy student. In these dialogues Socrates would expose the illogical thinking of the student and show him the correct way of thinking by asking pertinent questions. Typically, a Socratic dialogue starts with the student making some reasonable-sounding statement about some matter of philosophical interest and ends with the student making another statement along the lines of 'I see now, Socrates, that I was wrong when I said that...' and then summarising the arguments brought out in the dialogue. The dialogues of Plato make impressive reading for the aspiring CBT therapist but it must be remembered that in some ways Plato's task was easier than ours, not least because he supplied both the questions and answers whereas we therapists have control of the questions only – and our patients do not always answer as obligingly as Plato's philosophy students do!

A regular and frequent feature of CBT is the therapist's rephrasing, recapping and summarising of what the patient has said. This practice not only enables the therapist to clarify that he has understood what is going on but is also an essential part of the therapeutic process as it helps the patient to focus on the key issues. When rephrasing or summarising what the patient has said it is essential that the patient feels able to correct the therapist if that rephrasing is not accurate, so the therapist constantly questions along the lines 'Have I understood that properly?' or 'Have I got that right?' or 'I think we agreed that ... or could I put it more accurately?' etc. If the therapist has not understood or has expressed something inaccurately then he should take the responsibility for this himself – he should in no way imply that the patient was inarticulate or otherwise at fault.

As with most psychological therapies, good rapport and trust are essential ingredients of CBT. The therapist should have a positive regard for his patient and adopt a non-judgemental attitude to what he is told during therapy. He should be honest, warm and empathic and blame neither his patient nor himself when progress is slow.

The formation and maintenance of delusional beliefs

2

INTRODUCTION

Theories of mental illness have traditionally stressed either the biological causes (the so-called **medical model**) or the psychological causes (the so-called **psychosocial model**) and in the past there has been a tendency to compare and contrast these models as if they were contradictory and incompatible. This was inappropriate on both theoretical and practical grounds. We cannot separate off the psychological experience from the brain activity that produces it because they are different sides of the same coin; they are the subjective and objective descriptions of the same thing. Furthermore, it is now known that not only do the biochemistry and activity of the brain affect the psychological experience but also the psychological experience can affect the biochemistry and activity of the brain.

As far as schizophrenia is concerned, both biological abnormalities in the brain and stresses in the psychological environment are known to affect the onset and development of the symptoms, so at a clinical level it is more useful to regard the medical and psychosocial models of schizophrenia as complementary rather than alternatives. In practice, this means considering both the biological and psychological factors that might be relevant for a particular patient and seeking to produce a beneficial change by the use of biological and psychological treatments (e.g. medication and CBT respectively). In order to apply CBT to the symptoms of schizophrenia it is necessary to appreciate the role played by the underlying brain dysfunction, but it is not necessary to know exactly what that abnormality is or how it has arisen. Therefore, in this book we will not be considering the nature of the biological abnormalities associated with schizophrenia or the range of biological treatments that are currently available: interested readers are referred to standard psychiatric texts covering this area.

Since CBT is a psychological therapy we will be considering in some detail the psychological processes that are involved in the development and maintenance of delusions and hallucinations, taking into account not only the role played by abnormal functioning but also the important role played by the functioning of normal psychological processes. The psychological models presented in this chapter are based on current knowledge of normal psychological processing and of schizophrenia, but they have been heavily influenced by our clinical experience of using CBT strategies with people with schizophrenia.

There were two main reasons for developing these models as an aid to clinical practice, apart from the intrinsic fascination of trying to understand the very different forms that delusions and hallucinations can take in different people. The first reason was to provide the therapist with a framework within which he could structure his thinking about a particular delusion experienced by an individual patient and within which he could plan the appropriate strategies and treatment. The second reason was to provide the patient with a framework within which he could understand his symptoms and explain his experiences.

In order to make the models easy to comprehend and use with patients, they have been kept very simple, but inevitably this means that some relevant factors have had to be omitted. For this reason, they have been called working models, to reflect their practical use, rather than theoretical models. In practice, these models do seem to be very serviceable for most people's delusional beliefs but if an omitted factor (e.g. error in thinking) is particularly relevant for an individual patient then you can always put it in when adapting the model for his particular delusion.

The two principal models presented below are looking at slightly different aspects of the thinking and believing processes and so are not contradictory, but nevertheless it is suggested that you do not confuse your patient by trying to introduce more than one model at a time.

A WORKING MODEL FOR THE FORMATION AND MAINTENANCE OF DELUSIONAL BELIEFS

Adaptation of the general model for CBT

The model presented in Figure 1.4 (p. 15) to illustrate the formation and maintenance of new beliefs in non-psychotic people can be adapted to account for delusional beliefs by the simple addition of a 'psychotic activity' process, which is envisaged as some disturbance occurring at a physiological level within the brain and which can directly affect emotion/ mood state. This adaptation would suggest that whereas the process of belief formation is normally triggered by the situation that the person is in, in the case of delusional beliefs the process is triggered by a change in emotion or mood state. Because the mood state is driven by a biological disturbance rather than being a response to life experiences, it may be quite inappropriate to what is actually going on in the patient's life or the situation he is in, but it can trigger mood-congruent thoughts and hence beliefs that may seem inappropriate or even inexplicable to others. Once acquired, the delusional belief is maintained by the same psychological processes as are involved in the maintenance of normal beliefs (see Chapter 1, pp. 9–12).

The occurrence of a delusional mood state, often as a prelude to the onset of specific delusions, is well established in the psychiatric literature. The occurrence of a biologically driven mood state is also supported by our experience with longer term cognitive therapy with patients during relapse; in these cases patients have reported **feeling** as if such and such were so (e.g. that someone wanted to harm them) even though they were able to argue and know rationally that this was not so in fact.

Simplified model for the formation and maintenance of delusional beliefs

A simplified version of this model is presented in Figure 2.1. The inclusion of the basic biosocial system(s) into the model is optional and, at the present time, speculative, but it may be useful for explaining to patients why their illness produces the delusional feelings that it does. Our suggestion is that when the psychosis is active at a physiological level it may activate the neurological substrates of a basic biosocial system (e.g. defence or dominance) which is normally only activated by external events; this results in feelings and behaviours that are appropriate to that biosocial system. Because these systems are normally activated only by external events, it is appropriate that the brain should be programmed to seek for an external 'cause' for any activation of these systems, since it is only by locating the cause that the human animal can take appropriate action. Because the situations in which these systems are normally invoked are of such fundamental importance to the person's well-being, it is necessary for the brain to be able to come to a quick and decisive conclusion and so at this level it tends to work at an automatic level, jumping to conclusions in an all-or-nothing fashion. The seeking for the cause of the delusional mood state does not take place at a conscious level and so is not subject to rational analysis or thoughtful speculation.

The 'cause' that is found for the feelings will depend not only on the external situation but also on the person's beliefs and assumptions about the world; it may also be influenced by biased thinking, particularly the tendency to select evidence that is consistent with the person's prevailing mood state.

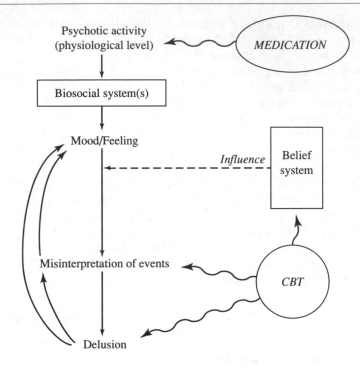

Fig. 2.1 Simplified working model for the formation and maintenance of a delusional belief.

The interpretation of events made by the brain may, in some circumstances, feel so convincing to the person concerned that it takes on the status of a belief without additional evidence being required and, being experienced as self-evidently true, will not therefore be subject to rational or critical reasoning ('It's obvious that ...'). Although delusional beliefs can appear quite suddenly in this way, they may also be built up more slowly, as a result of an accumulation of evidence provided by the repeated occurrence of delusional mood-driven misinterpretations.

Example of the model in action

1. A patient is sitting in his room at home with his wife and a CPN who has visited to give him his depot injection. He has a psychotic episode which leads him to feel threatened.
2. Like all human beings, he will be predisposed to see other people as more likely sources of threat than inanimate objects such as the

furniture in his room, so the 'source' of threat will crystallise around either his wife or the CPN. If he has a good relationship with his wife and believes her to be caring and loving it is unlikely that the fear will attach itself to her but if he knows the CPN less well and perhaps has some reservations about his injections, then it is likely that the CPN will be perceived as the source of threat. Thus the first misperception of events, driven by his feeling of threat but influenced by his existing beliefs about his wife, the CPN and the injections, has occurred.

3. Once a belief about the CPN wanting to harm him has emerged then it will influence his interpretation of subsequent events so that they conform to and thereby confirm the belief. For example, supposing the CPN visits next day to offer to take him to the shops. The offer is kindly meant but, believing that the CPN wishes him harm, it is inter-preted by the patient as a plot to get him away from the safety of his home and the protection of his wife. This interpretation will increase his feelings of paranoia and confirm his delusional belief that the CPN wants to harm him. The self-confirming circle has been brought into effect.

4. The belief about the CPN will be further strengthened if the psychotic episode triggers more paranoid feelings, because once the delusion about the CPN has been established then these subsequent paranoid feelings are likely also to be associated with the CPN.

5. Once the belief that the CPN wants to harm him has been firmly established then the self-confirming belief circles will act so as to maintain it even after the psychotic episode has finished. The patient now has a chronic delusion that can only be overturned if he is presented with overwhelming evidence and argument to refute it.

Implications of the model for treatment

There are a number of implications for the type and effectiveness of treatment that follow directly from this model.

1. CBT can be used to break the cycle maintaining the delusion, by modifying the misinterpretation of events that serve to reinforce the delusional belief and/or by direct modification of the delusional belief itself.

2. Because of the influence that pre-existing non-psychotic beliefs may have on the way that the delusional mood/feeling state is made sense of, i.e. on the particular form that the delusion takes, it may be appro-priate to undertake CBT on these pre-existing beliefs as part of the overall treatment package.

3. When the neuropsychotic activity is quiescent and therefore not producing a delusional mood state, then it should be possible for CBT to completely eliminate the delusional belief and hence the unpleasant feelings associated with it.

4. However, when the psychosis is active, even though CBT may be able to hold the delusional belief at bay by challenging the misinterpretation of events and even the delusion itself, the unpleasant feelings produced by the psychosis will remain and this will increase vulnerability to mood-congruent delusional thoughts. At this time, the optimal therapeutic position for the patient is that he is able to make the distinction 'I feel as if ... but I know really that...'.

5. Being able to use reason to counter the influence of the mood and the delusional thoughts when the psychosis is active has two clear benefits. First, it limits the duration of the unpleasant feelings to when the psychosis is active so that when the psychosis dies away at a physiological level it does not leave behind an established delusional belief that would continue to give problems. Second, it may enable the patient to act on what he knows rather than what he feels and thereby enable him to put coping strategies into effect.

6. Even if a delusional belief has been effectively eradicated, it may re-emerge if the psychosis becomes active again because the mood state that was responsible for its development has occurred again. This being so, treatment should not only deal with the present situation but should also provide the patient with CBT strategies that he can use to counter the delusional belief if and when it recurs in the future.

7. Antipsychotic medication can prevent the occurrence and reinforcement of delusional beliefs by preventing the biological disturbance that drives the delusional mood state.

Note that for many patients, medication is able to eliminate established delusional beliefs without the aid of CBT. This is because once the mood/feeling that drives the delusion has been eliminated, then the conflicting evidence from everyday events, influenced by the patient's other beliefs, is enough to change the delusion. In effect, the CBT part of the treatment has occurred naturally.

Example of the model in action

In the example given above, CBT would be used as follows.

1. To change the misinterpretation of events that are reinforcing the delusion about the CPN. For example, one goal would be to change the patient's interpretation of the CPN's offer to take him to the shops to the more likely explanation that he intended this to be helpful for the patient as part of his rehabilitation programme.

2. To change the underlying delusion about the CPN. This would involve a direct challenge to his belief that the CPN wanted to harm him, the goal being for him to believe that the CPN was trying to help him and had his best interests at heart. This would be done by using some of the strategies described in Chapter 9.

3. To alter the belief about medication doing more harm than good. If the patient believes medication is bad for him, it is not unreasonable for him to conclude that the person who gives him the medication does not have his best interests at heart and may even wish him harm. The aim would be to change his belief about medication to a belief that medication is generally beneficial for him, though acknowledging that there are probably some unwanted side effects.

4. Whilst the psychosis is active at a biological level, medication will be needed to control the paranoid feelings that result directly from his illness. If this is not possible, then the best position may be for him to be able to reason 'I feel as if the CPN wants to harm me but I know he doesn't really because...'. 'These feelings are caused by my illness and it might help if I...'.

THE TWO-ROUTE MODEL OF RESPONDING

The two-route model of responding, illustrated in Figure 2.2, gives an alternative way of explaining to patients why they might feel convinced that something was true even though there was no apparent evidence to back it up, why those feelings might be misleading and how CBT strategies could help to correct them. It can often be used at an earlier stage of therapy than the models for the development and maintenance of the delusions because it does not carry the same suggestion of underlying brain dysfunction and illness and so is less likely to bring about unwanted insight or to be experienced by the patient as a challenge to his delusional beliefs.

The two-route model illustrates two ways we have of responding to a situation. It should be noted that this response may be in the form of a thought as well as an action. The lower route corresponds to the lower level, automatic responses that result from the functioning of the more primitive, animal parts of our brain concerned with our more basic needs such as safety and our position in society. Because this route is concerned with our survival and well-being it has to be capable of responding quickly and so it is characterised by a single, rapid, all-or-nothing type of response. For this route, jumping to conclusions is a virtue, not a vice, because it enables fast, decisive conclusions to be drawn and action to be taken. This route is also geared to operate on a better-safe-than-sorry principle since, for example, it is better for an animal to take protective

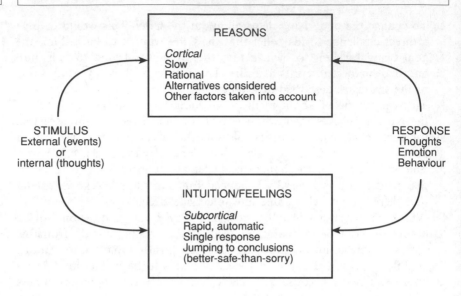

Fig. 2.2 Two-route model of thinking/responding.

action when there is no threat than to fail to take such action when that threat exists. In order to prompt rapid action the conclusion reached must feel as if it is absolutely correct; the animal cannot afford to dither and so the conclusion is accompanied by a sense of conviction in its correctness. If this sense of conviction is very strong, then the conclusion, reached without any conscious thought or awareness on the part of the person concerned, may be experienced subjectively as an intuition.

The higher level route of responding uses the rational thinking abilities of the more advanced parts of our brain. Previous memories may be tapped as alternative interpretations are considered and alternative courses of action and the possible consequences of those actions are thought through. This route is able to handle probabilities and to weigh up the different options before coming to a final conclusion. Because of the greater range and depth of the thinking via this route it takes longer to respond but is likely to be more accurate in its analysis of the situation. We are consciously aware of much of the thinking that goes on in this route and to a large extent we are able to control the direction it takes.

In normal situations both routes of responding operate, the subcortical route producing a rapid response that is then tempered or modified by the slower rational thinking of the cortical route. For example, if a balloon burst whilst you were in the supermarket your immediate response is likely to be to drop your head down and hunch your shoulders into a protective position, but this defensive posture will be quickly dropped when you look behind and realise that the sound was only a balloon bursting.

The rapid response does not have to involve a physical action; it can be, and indeed very often is, a thought. In normal situations this rapid thought is then checked and weighed up against the deliberations of the slower, rational route. For example, you are lying in a hospital bed when a rather attractive nurse/doctor smiles warmly at you. The thought flashes into your mind that he/she is sexually attracted to you and is seeking to start a relationship. It will not take long for your slower, rational route to come up with the conclusion that the nurse/doctor is most probably merely being kind.

The two-route model explains how we respond in normal situations and is not specific to delusional thoughts or delusional beliefs. What may happen in schizophrenia is that the lower route is relatively more active and/or the conclusions reached by this route are accompanied by an unusually strong sense of conviction about their correctness. Be that as it may, we have found that patients find this model easy to understand and to relate to their own experiences. It gives them a reason why their sense of certainty about things might be misleading and is useful for explaining what the strategies of the CBT treatment are seeking to achieve in helping to monitor the lower route and to strengthen the higher, more reliable way of thinking.

In some cases, it appears that delusional beliefs may develop directly from automatic thoughts, without involving events in the exterior world. In such a case it seems that the automatic thought is not subject to the normal filtering and selection of ideas that occurs in the conscious brain but, as part of the psychotic process, is directly invested with confirmed-belief status. This could account for the occurrence of delusional beliefs that are quite bizarre and unrelated to the real world. The process involved may be similar to that seen with LSD, where subjects under the influence of the drug may receive sudden revelations of 'profound truths' (e.g. the world is made of cheese) which are then held with complete conviction despite their factual absurdity. The whole question of when and why the brain confers confirmed-belief status on particular ideas is a very interesting one, though at this time we can only speculate about it. We saw in Chapter 1 why it is functional for our beliefs to be held with a greater sense of certainty than the evidence would perhaps warrant, because this means that we no longer have to seek and weigh up evidence as to their correctness and also it enables us to use these beliefs without hesitation. This suggests that there must be some function within the brain that decides when probability is converted to a feeling of certainty. It is interesting to speculate that this may be the 'normal' process that is inappropriately triggered in schizophrenia in the formation of these bizarre delusional beliefs.

HOW COGNITIVE THERAPY WORKS ON DELUSIONS

We saw in Chapter 1 how the belief change that occurs in cognitive therapy comes about as the result of a new, incompatible belief being established which then overlays the old belief rather than completely eradicating it. The same thing happens with CBT with delusions. Given the amount of work done in CBT to target specific delusions, one might intuitively expect that should a relapse occur in the future then a different delusion would develop, albeit on the same theme as the original delusion, because so many reasons **not** to believe the original delusion had been amassed. Certainly, when I first started modifying delusions I shared my colleagues' concern that another delusion might just take the place of the one we had taken such trouble to modify and so treatment would be endless. However, we have found in practice that substitute delusions do not occur in this way; when there is a relapse, it is the same delusions, in the same form, that tend to recur.

This fact is good news for long-term therapy because it means that the specific strategies developed during CBT treatment to target the particular delusions that the patient has will also be appropriate for longer term use. The patient can be prepared for a relapse with a tailor-made set of specific CBT strategies.

The down-side of the fact that the new beliefs established during CBT do not completely eradicate the delusional beliefs is that the person will always be potentially vulnerable to a reactivation of these delusional beliefs in the future, should the conditions be right. Patients who make a full recovery as a result of medication and/or the passage of time are potentially more likely to re-acquire their old delusional beliefs than patients who have also received CBT because they do not have the CBT skills to detect and counter the delusional ideas as they are re-emerging. Because of this potential for delusional beliefs to be reactivated in the future, CBT has a role to play even if the patient is quite well again by the time you meet him and he no longer believes his delusions to be true. At this time, work can be done to strengthen his current incompatible, non-delusional beliefs and also to provide him with other specific cognitive strategies to detect and counter the delusional beliefs should they recur in the future.

CBT is generally given as an adjunctive treatment to medication, to treat the residual symptoms and problems that remain after the best possible medication regime has been found (see pp. 49–50). Other things being equal, it is recommended that CBT treatment is given to the patient when he is at his least psychotic. There are three main reasons for this. First, CBT is a time-consuming treatment, both for the patient and therapist, so it is not time effective to use CBT unnecessarily. Second, the CBT will be easier and progress faster if the patient is relatively well, both because rapport is likely to be easier to retain and also because less firmly held delusions are easier to challenge. Third, CBT will stand a better chance of success if the delusional mood and feelings are not being constantly refreshed by the illness. Whilst the delusional feelings are being activated at a biological level the delusional beliefs will be reinforced both by the distorting effect that the delusional feelings will have on the interpretation of everyday events and also by the fact that the delusional beliefs are mood congruent. When the psychosis is no longer active at a biological level the CBT has to combat only the cognitive processes that are maintaining the delusional belief and not the effects of the biologically driven delusional feelings as well.

The exception to the above recommendation is with first-episode patients, because evidence is emerging from studies to suggest that early CBT intervention can help to prevent the establishment of delusional beliefs, leading to faster and more complete recovery. If this proves to be so, then getting to work with first-episode patients before medication has had time to take effect may be beneficial for the long term, even though it is likely to be more difficult and to take longer in the short term if the patient is distracted and/or thought disordered.

The ways in which CBT works on delusions can be summarised as follows.

1. Cognitive behavioural therapy works by strengthening the reasoning/rational side of the person to argue against and thereby to influence the intuitional/feelings side.
2. It encourages the patient to make the split between 'I feel ... but I know ...'. This is particularly important for when the psychosis is active because at this time the feelings will continue to some degree, however good the rational arguments against them might be.
3. It encourages the patient to act on the 'I know ...' rather than on the 'I feel ...'. In other words, it enables the patient to select a behaviour that will reduce rather than increase the strength of the delusional belief. For example, a young man who developed paranoid delusions about the nurses when unwell would isolate himself in his room, thereby providing more evidence that they were not concerned about him. Following CBT, he was able to detect and identify the re-emergence of these ideas as his psychosis fluctuated and, by using reason to counter the paranoid feelings whilst they were still mild, he was able to put into effect the previously discovered coping strategy of going to talk to the nurses. Their friendly response provided immediate feedback and evidence against the paranoid thoughts and thereby prevented the full-blown delusion from developing.
4. Having insight and being able to argue rationally against a delusional belief will lessen the impact that the delusional thoughts would

otherwise have on emotions and behaviour. It will also help to prevent the development of secondary delusional beliefs. For example, in the case mentioned above, being able to produce evidence that the nursing staff felt kindly towards him prevented this paranoid patient developing a secondary delusional belief that the medication the nursing staff were giving him might be harming him.

5. CBT is more effective and progresses faster the less actively psychotic the patient, so when used as an adjunct to medication it is often appropriate to wait until the patient has settled down on his medication before starting the CBT.

Talking to people with schizophrenia

3

DISCUSSING DELUSIONS AND HALLUCINATIONS

Good rapport and trust are essential

Unlike other conditions, where people come to a therapist seeking help for an identified and recognised problem, people with schizophrenia may have no insight into their condition, no recognition that they have a problem that could be helped and therefore little reason to engage in a series of therapy sessions. In such cases, good rapport with the therapist is essential because the relationship the patient has with you may be the only reason for him to attend your sessions, at least in the earlier stages of therapy. Good rapport and trust are also essential when you start challenging the delusional beliefs. Having the inaccuracies of one's beliefs exposed is generally not a pleasant experience and so it is important that your patient is confident that you respect him and that he does not experience your questioning as a personal attack or as being critical of him in any way. Paranoid patients are particularly likely to interpret challenging questions as a personal threat and so you must have a correspondingly good relationship with a paranoid patient in order to counter any paranoid ideas about you that may arise when you are doing therapy.

Because the therapeutic relationship is so important for the success of CBT with schizophrenia, you may need to spend quite a lot of time building up rapport and trust, both before you start active CBT work and to maintain the relationship whilst therapy is progressing. It is not uncommon for me to spend weeks (and occasionally even months) building up rapport before attempting to do any direct belief modifica-tion work, and after embarking on a CBT programme I usually spend around half the session talking about things that are not directly related to the CBT programme except in that it is helping to maintain the therapeutic relationship. With less ill people who have more insight you can start the modification work more quickly, and once your patient understands what the therapy is seeking to achieve then the modification work is itself rewarding for him and more time can be spent on it within the session.

Provide a safe environment

It is known that in the animal kingdom social animals are more likely to explore or undertake other 'risky' behaviours if they are not alone; being with one of their own kind not only affects behaviour but also produces measurable biochemical changes in the brain. This effect can also be seen to operate in everyday human life. For example, most people feel safer at night if there is someone else in the house than if they are on their own (Why is it that it is only when one is alone that the stairs creak, the pipes make sinister noises and there are unexplained bangs from downstairs?). This sense of safety does not seem to be due only to the fact that another person could provide additional defence in case of intrusion or other emergency, since it also operates to some extent if that other person is a young child or infirm elderly person who could not provide any protection in case of danger.

It is thought that a good interpersonal relationship between patient and therapist is important for CBT in schizophrenia because the sense of safety that it provides enables the patient to explore some of his frightening experiences and beliefs in a way that he would not be able to do on his own. Paradoxically, although it may be harder to build up a trusting relationship with a paranoid patient, the therapeutic relationship may be a particularly important component of the therapy in these cases.

Familiar surroundings also tend to create feelings of safety, so where possible you should see your patient for therapy in the same room. It is worth paying some attention to the layout and furnishing of the room in order to create a warm and comfortable atmosphere. Not only will a relaxing environment make the sessions more pleasant for your patients, it may also help them to feel safer. Although you may have standard-issue furnishings you can still make a big difference to the atmosphere by adding a rug, potted plants, ornaments, etc.

If you are seeing your patient in the community, you may have the choice between seeing him in his home or on health service premises. It is probably better not to see your patient in his own home unless you are already visiting him there (e.g. as his CPN) or unless he is unwilling to make the journey to see you anywhere else. 'Home' is good from the point of view of being a familiar and safe environment for the patient but being in the role of visitor to the patient's home can conflict with your role as therapist in the therapeutic relationship. Needless to say, if there is any risk of a violent reaction to your visit or to your questioning, then you should not see the patient alone in his home.

Empathise with the patient's feelings

A key to working with people with schizophrenia is to have empathy for their feelings and emotions and to express this empathy in words and gestures. However, it will not always be possible to understand exactly what your patient feels and in some cases you may be quite unable even to imagine what he might be feeling. Have you ever tried to imagine what an extra 'sense' might be like, other than in terms of seeing, hearing, touch, etc.? For most of us it is quite impossible to imagine what this would be like because we can only think in terms of the senses that we have experienced. Similarly, since some of the feelings and experiences produced by the psychotic brain are likely to be outside the realm of our non-psychotic experiences, they will also be beyond our powers of imagination.

At the best of times our human vocabulary is relatively imprecise and non-specific when it comes to describing internal subjective experiences and this may impose yet another restriction on communication. Thus the patient may have no words with which to adequately describe his psychotic experiences, even if we were capable of understanding what he was trying to convey. It may also be impossible to understand what the patient is feeling if his explanation is in such idiosyncratic or thought-disordered language that it makes no obvious sense to you (e.g. 'It's the transmigration of the intergalactic figures, sitting still'). Despite these problems in communicating feeling and experiences, even if you cannot understand or imagine what your patient is feeling, you can ask him whether the experience is pleasant or unpleasant, frightening or comforting, important or insignificant, etc. so that you can have an empathic appreciation at least at this very basic level.

Perhaps the most important thing to remember for empathy is that it makes no difference to how your patient feels whether or not his beliefs or fears are actually true in the 'real' world; this is so for all of us, of course, not just for people with schizophrenia. For example, if a police-woman were to knock at your door now to inform you that your partner, child or parent had been killed in a car crash you would probably be very upset. The fact that you will be told in an hour's time that there had been a terrible mistake, that your loved one was actually quite safe and well, would not in any way affect how you feel now, since you have no way of knowing that this would happen in the future. Similarly, for the person with schizophrenia, the fact that his voice will not succeed in carrying out its threat to kill him next year or the fact that he will not actually die from poisoning in the future will do nothing to relieve his feelings and fears **now**. So as far as empathising with the feelings is concerned, the same empathy is appropriate whether the belief is true in fact or not, since the intensity of the feelings will be the same.

A simple way of triggering empathy in the clinical situation is to imagine that the belief or fear were actually true and that it affected you rather than your patient – how would that make you feel? What commonly happens in this situation is that we take into account our own beliefs about reality when we evaluate the patient's feelings and temper our empathy accordingly; this is something that we have to be constantly alert not to do. An easy test to check if you are doing this is to ask yourself 'If this were really happening to the patient, would I feel the same way about what he is going through?'. If the answer is 'no' then you are not empathising completely with the patient's feelings in his situation. An example from clinical practice to illustrate this point was a lady I saw recently who believed that nursing staff had operated on her in the night and removed her body organs. Whilst I appreciated that she was recalling a very unpleasant experience, I was aware on applying the above test that my concern and expression of concern were not what they would have been if she had really been operated on in this way.

It may be particularly difficult to sustain empathy with delusions that are obviously incorrect, when they recur frequently. This was brought home to me many years ago when I attended my first case conference on a continuing care ward and heard a patient describe his intense fear that his voice would carry out its threat to cut off his head in the next day or so. I was deeply moved by his distress and was surprised, therefore, when the rest of the team calmly discussed his progress and opted to wait for another week before reviewing his medication. And neither does being aware of this effect make one immune to it. One of my own patients would wake up every morning believing she was going to die later that day and seek me out to tell me of her fears; despite being aware of the 'fading empathy' effect, it was difficult to be as patient and concerned at the end of a fortnight of interruptions as it had been at the beginning. It is almost as if we expect the patient to realise that because these things keep happening they cannot really be true and therefore that they should not really be upsetting; but of course the very essence of these delusional beliefs is that they do retain their immediacy and conviction even over long periods. The lesson I have learnt over the years is that with recurring delusional beliefs it is particularly important to remind myself to imagine the situation afresh from time to time, to feel again what it must be like to believe these things to be true and about to happen, and to remember how I felt when the patient first told me of these terrible things.

It may also be difficult to feel spontaneous empathy for a belief that appears impossible or even ridiculous, for example one patient who believed that a shark might come and eat her on the ward. Again, the key to feeling empathy is to imagine that the impossible has happened and that the belief has come true. Alternatively, you can try imagining a similar but possible situation in order to feel what it must be like to believe as the patient does; for example, in the above case imagining that you were swimming in the sea and suddenly realising there were sharks around.

There may be a temptation to try to joke the patient out of a 'ridiculous' belief, a temptation that should always be resisted; not only would the attempt be unsuccessful, it would also be grossly insensitive and unkind. Humour does have a part to play in therapy and, indeed, it can be an important part, but this must be led by the patient himself. Even when your patient has developed enough insight to be able to laugh about one of his previously held delusional ideas you should always acknowledge and re-express your empathy with the feelings that this generated at the time; for example, 'I suppose looking back on it now it does seem a funny idea, the shark flapping its tail in its attempts to move across the open field and then trying to climb up the flight of stairs to your ward, because you're absolutely right when you say that no shark could live or move out of water..., but nevertheless it must have been a terrifying thought when it seemed as if it could actually happen'.

Similarly, it can be particularly important to re-express empathy with your patient's feelings immediately after he has made the intellectual step of rejecting his delusional belief. Your empathy will signal your recognition that his current understanding in no way diminishes the distress he felt when he believed his delusion to be true and that he was not foolish for believing or feeling the way he did at that time. You can also use this opportunity to summarise and rephrase what the patient has discovered, highlighting the fact that believing something to be true does not mean that it is true in fact, a key insight for work with delusions. For example, 'From the work we've done it does look as if you were wrong when you thought your sister had tried to poison you; I am sure you are right when you say that she wouldn't visit you and buy you presents if she hated you enough to want to poison you, but it must have been really frightening when that idea came into your mind and seemed so true, because you didn't know then that it was going to turn out not to be true'.

Be aware of your own beliefs and prejudices about the symptoms and label of schizophrenia

One of the approaches used to help patients see that they themselves are not weird or peculiar because they have weird or peculiar thoughts and experiences is for staff to share their own strange experiences with the patients (see pp. 84 and 179). This is done in order to demonstrate that most people's brains are capable of producing odd and inaccurate experiences of the world and therefore that the patient is not set apart from the rest of human kind because of his ideas or experiences. When doing this exercise you should notice if you feel any hesitation about sharing your own odd ideas and experiences with your patient or with your colleagues or an urge to explain why you had them (e.g. I was very tired, I had been under a lot of stress). These are very common reactions but interesting in that they indicate that even in apparently well-informed and accepting mental health professionals, such as ourselves, there is still a stigma attached to mental illness such that we do not want to risk our patients or colleagues drawing any wrong conclusions about us or our experiences! But why does it matter if one of your colleagues thinks you have had a genuine psychotic experience or thinks that you are showing some of the signs of schizophrenia?

Believe the patient until proved otherwise or at least suspend your disbelief

If you were to tell me that I am not a trained clinical psychologist, I would probably conclude that you are either ignorant, stupid or deliberately trying to wind me up. If a number of people repeated the same thing and threatened to take me into hospital for stating what I know to be the truth, then I might quite reasonably conclude that there was some nasty conspiracy going on. It is not surprising if people with schizophrenia react similarly when their beliefs, which they know to be true with as much certainty as I know I am a clinical psychologist, are refuted. Openly denying the truth of the patient's beliefs, describing them as delusions and attributing them to an illness, is probably the most common reason for poor rapport between staff and patient. At best, frank disbelief may indicate to the patient with no insight that you have failed to understand how things really are for him and at worst it may imply some wilful and malevolent reason for your denial. For the sake of building rapport it is better to believe your patient until you can prove otherwise; and this latter does not mean until you, the therapist, can prove to your own satisfaction that the belief is not true but rather until you and the patient working together can prove otherwise to your mutual satisfaction. This does not mean that you have to believe that your patient is definitely correct or even probably correct, only that you reserve the possibility that the patient could be correct, i.e. you suspend your disbelief.

In practice, it is nearly always possible to be genuine in your suspension of disbelief about a delusion providing you are humble enough to acknowledge that you cannot justify absolute certainty for most of your own beliefs, including those against which you are judging the patient's delusional beliefs. For example, a patient of mine believes she is inhabited by a ghost. Whilst I believe that ghosts do not exist and that symptoms such as those of my patient can be caused by a brain disorder, if I am strictly honest I have to admit that I cannot be absolutely certain that I am right or absolutely certain that my patient is wrong, so I have to allow for the possibility (albeit remote) that the patient could be inhabited by a ghost, as she claims. Similarly, no-one can be absolutely certain that Martians do not exist, that Hitler cannot be reincarnated, that God does not send messages in the shapes of clouds, etc.

When first introduced to this way of working, some people are concerned that, in talking to their patient about his delusional beliefs as if they could be true, they are somehow being hypocritical, that instead they should be informing him firmly and authoritatively that they are just delusions. I have never understood why the therapeutic ideal of honesty has been interpreted as brutal frankness and why this should supersede the therapeutic ideals of respect and regard for the patient and sensitivity for his feelings, especially as we do not respond this way to other people we meet in our everyday lives, in social and work situations. For example, if I meet someone at a party who tells me of some strange course of exercises she is attending in order to help her get pregnant, I do not feel obliged to tell her that I think it will not work and that she is wasting her money, and if a colleague at work has clearly misunderstood a research paper I do not feel that I ought to tell her that she has completely missed the point (especially if it is a senior colleague!). Similarly, if a friend is comforted by the messages from her dead husband given to her by a medium, I do not feel compelled to tell her that it is a load of rubbish. So why do we feel the need to tell our patients that what they believe so profoundly to be true is a load of rubbish? Because, like it or not, that is exactly what we are telling them when we inform them so dogmatically that their ideas and beliefs are delusions.

It can be a difficult moment if your patient asks you directly if you believe as he does, so you should have already considered how you will answer such a question in order to avoid hesitating in your response. In practice, I have found it rare for patients to ask me directly if I believe as they do. Perhaps this is because patients are reluctant to put the issue to the test; having experienced people dismissing what they have said in the past, they may be reluctant to risk losing the support and interest of someone who does take them seriously and who is prepared to investigate what is going on. However, if you are asked the direct question, then of course you should answer it honestly; certainly it is unlikely to help progress in the long term if you support the delusion to the extent of saying that you also believe it to be true. However, whether you tell the whole truth in these circumstances is a matter of clinical judgement and how much of your own views you share with your patient is likely to change as therapy progresses. For example, if your patient's enquiry has come at a later stage of therapy, when he is re-evaluating the likelihood of his delusional belief and is genuinely asking for your opinion as part of that re-evaluation, then you should tell the whole truth as you understand it. On the other hand, if the enquiry occurs early on in therapy, when it is more in the nature of a check that you are not like everybody else in dismissing the beliefs as 'nonsense' or 'illness', then it is appropriate to be honest in less precise terms. For example, when first asked this question by the woman who was inhabited by a ghost, I told her that I had no way of knowing for certain – I was only able to go on her explanation of what was going on but that I had no reason to disbelieve what she told me. When this question was repeated several sessions later, when rapport was stronger, I was able to introduce a stronger note of doubt by noting that the doctors believed her symptoms were due to an illness and so, not having had the patient's experiences myself, how could I be sure which explanation was correct?

Whilst you are keeping open the possibility that your patient's interpretation of events just might be correct, you should of course be speculating about other possible explanations for the patient's experiences and other possible interpretations of situations and events, because these speculations will guide your questioning. For example, are the neighbours next door really shouting abuse at the patient or has he misinterpreted a family row or their noisy conversations, or is he hearing 'voices' that have nothing to do with quiet, polite neighbours next door? You can then ask your patient the relevant questions to help clarify which of these alternatives might be correct. In the above example, you might ask 'What time of day/night did this happen?', 'Where were you when this happened?', 'Could you see them when they are doing this?', etc. In my own clinical experience I have found it very rare for patients to imagine events that have no basis in fact at all, although their perception and interpretation of the events can be grossly distorted. Therefore, I usually find it helpful to approach even situations that clearly cannot have happened in fact with a view to trying to work out what 'really' happened. In the example just mentioned, if the patient reported that he could see the neighbours in the garden at the time of their shouted abuse then I would be confident that they had been there, but I would reserve my judgement about his report that they looked threatening or that they were being abusive to him until there was more evidence to indicate whether or not this was likely behaviour from the neighbours.

We believe that suspending disbelief is a key feature for successful CBT with people with schizophrenia, not only because respecting the patient's point of view helps to build up rapport but also because keeping an open mind will enable you to discuss the patient's beliefs and experiences in a natural and genuine way that is not possible if you have prejudged the issue as an open-and-shut case. Furthermore, this approach allows you to explore the beliefs and experiences with your patient in a genuine joint exercise. The only time it is not appropriate to suspend your disbelief is when your patient has an unpleasant belief and would rather have your reassurance that you do not believe it to be true than your willingness to consider his belief with an open mind (see Chapter 6).

Talk to the patient naturally

Believing what the patient tells you, or at least believing that it is possible, will lead you to ask questions naturally, using words that do not imply disbelief. If you are finding it difficult to suspend your disbelief it may help if you imagine that a friend is telling you of these experiences. How would you respond? What questions would you ask?

When talking to patients about their delusions and hallucinations, a mistake that is commonly made is to use the word 'think' when asking the patient about something that he has told you is fact. The questions 'What made you think...' and 'How did you know...?' are essentially the same in that they are seeking the same information, but the 'think' question implies doubt about the patient's conclusions whereas the 'know' question does not. 'What happened...?' may elicit useful information without questioning its veracity.

It is important to recognise that we also communicate what we think and mean in ways apart from the words we actually use. Tone of voice is important in indicating how we feel about what we are saying whilst the inflexion in our voice and the stress that we put on words can significantly affect the meaning that is conveyed. These aspects of our speech occur spontaneously and automatically and so are very difficult to control consciously. Thus it is difficult not to 'leak' what you really believe when you talk to a patient. Genuinely suspending your disbelief is the best way to automatically control the language and intonation that you use.

Avoid collusion – agree to differ

Traditionally, mental health workers have been taught not to 'collude' with delusions and hallucinations. Whilst this is a sound principle, the way in which the term has been interpreted has had a most unfortunate impact on patient care. Many people working with schizophrenia have been led to think that they should avoid talking to patients about these experiences altogether, or that if delusional beliefs do come up in their discussions then they should advise the patient kindly but firmly that they are nothing more than symptoms of an illness and therefore should be disregarded. Imagine that you have just been told that you have a fatal illness that will kill you within weeks; how would you feel if the people you told ignored you or tried to change the subject to tomorrow's lunch menu or offered you a game of ping-pong. Angry? Rejected? So how must patients feel when, for example, they are worried that someone is trying to poison them or are frightened by threats from their voices and they find that members of staff will not talk to them about it? Presumably much the same as if these terrible things were really happening to them and people were indifferent to their suffering. I have always thought it must be particularly galling for patients that someone who has not been where they have been and has not experienced what they have experienced, nevertheless has the temerity to dismiss their version and explanation of events in favour of his own.

It is not helpful for therapy in the long run for the therapist to actively confirm a delusional belief, either directly or indirectly, as this may be taken as firm and authoritative evidence in its support. For example, one of our patients who believed she had an immaculate conception had been told some years earlier by her doctor to take her medication 'because it will be good for your baby'. It is not surprising that she used this later as key evidence to support her belief that her current doctors were just pretending when they said they did not believe in her pregnancy. Nevertheless, not colluding does not mean that you should not talk to your patient about these issues and take them seriously. Listening to the patient and respecting his opinions about what is going on will not strengthen his conviction in his delusional belief – he already believes it to be true, probably despite many people telling him he is wrong – but being perceived as an interested and caring person, who has not prejudged the issues, will put you in a position to ask questions and work therapeutically with your patient.

Especially as rapport develops, you can afford to hold a different point of view to that of your patient or to express your doubt without it damaging the therapeutic relationship providing there is an agreement to differ, much as one may agree to differ with a friend about a political issue where this could lead to arguments. But it is important that if you do agree to differ with your patient you in no way imply (or even believe!) that because you are the therapist your point of view is more likely to be correct than your patient's.

Meet with the patient before reading his medical notes

For a number of reasons I recommend meeting with patients before finding out details about the case. First, this will enable you to get a clearer picture of how things seem to the patient and what his priorities are. If you see a patient without knowing his background or history it is surprising how often you emerge from that first session feeling confused about what has been happening and unsure why he is in hospital. I think this feeling of confusion is useful because it mirrors the patient's feelings of confusion. Secondly, seeing the patient before reading his notes stops you prejudging the issues. Are the neighbours really that unpleasant? Are they really shouting abuse over the back fence and taking the patient's milk from his doorstep? Without reading the notes you cannot attribute these experiences to fact or paranoia because you just do not know and as a result you are likely to be more open-minded about them. Furthermore, there is an unfortunate tendency to attribute everything to the mental illness once this has been diagnosed: it is as if once you have a diagnosis of schizophrenia people cannot be unpleasant to you any more, you cannot lose your temper because someone has been irritating you, etc. Knowing that fellow professionals have attributed the patient's experiences to delusions and hallucinations will inevitably influence your own evaluation, so it is better not to know their views before you have had a chance to form your own. Thirdly, being unable to prejudge the issues is beneficial not only for empathy (it is easier to be empathic about something that might have happened than something you know is imagination) but also because it will lead you to ask the appropriate questions naturally. As you seek to get the information you need to decide whether the patient's interpretation of events corresponds to reality or not, you will also be gathering the information you will need later should belief modification be appropriate.

The fourth advantage of not reading the patient's notes before you see him is that if he cannot recall what has happened when he became ill or why he came into hospital then you can offer to find this out from his notes in order to discuss it with him, and this offer is a genuine one. Patients often have a poor recall of the events that brought them into hospital. This is not just reluctance to recall unpleasant events and experiences but is likely to reflect a genuine memory problem, presumably because the brain is not efficient at storing memories when it is suffering from a psychotic disturbance. Patients who are puzzled about why they are in hospital are often quite surprised but generally pleased that you should offer to find these things out for them. Having obtained the information in this way, you will then be able to share and discuss it with your patient, for example, 'It says in the notes that ... Is that how you recall it happening?'.

If you are unable to elicit the patient's delusional beliefs in the normal way during assessment or therapy then you may have to take the lead of introducing the topic to the patient. It is easier to adopt a neutral stance with respect to information gleaned from the hospital notes than to information given to you by a colleague. For example, 'When I was looking through your old hospital notes I noticed that they mentioned there was a time when you were having a feeling in your head, like an evil spirit was talking to you. That sounds really unpleasant. What happened, can you remember?'. If the patient is adamant that nothing like that ever happened you can retreat to the position that 'The notes seem to have got it wrong', which is less damaging to multidisciplinary team working than concluding that a colleague seems to have got it wrong.

Don't push too hard – be prepared to back off

Although we talk about 'challenging' delusions, this is nearly always done very gently, chipping or nibbling away at the belief rather than attacking it with a head-on assault. Directly challenging the delusion in a confrontational way is rarely correct. At best it risks damaging rapport and at worst it may actually strengthen conviction in the delusional belief. This paradoxical effect, whereby strong opposition may strengthen rather than weaken a belief, is not peculiar to delusional beliefs but applies to any firmly held belief. We must all have had the experience of having one of our treasured political or moral beliefs questioned by someone with opposing views. Did you find yourself suddenly doubting your beliefs or did you just become more extreme as you mustered more arguments to support your view?

The patient's conviction in a delusion may vary from time to time, so sensitivity is required to know how far to discuss and question a delusion at any one time. Particularly where the psychosis is fluctuating, the therapist must be prepared to make progress on one session only to find that what was agreed during one session is refuted the next. Because of this potential for people's insight and delusions to fluctuate, you should be particularly careful when starting a session by recapping the previous session's work. Asking the patient general questions about how he has been since the last session should give you a good indication of his current mental state and if you feel this has deteriorated then your recapping should be particularly tentative, e.g. 'Can you remember what we were talking about last week...?' or 'I'm not sure if I have remembered correctly but I think you were saying something last session about ... Am I right?'.

Summary

When talking to people with schizophrenia try to see and feel the situation from their point of view. If you can do this, everything else will follow naturally – your empathy, your expression of this empathy, your questions and the way you express your questions. Whilst part of you is keeping an enquiring scepticism about your patient's interpretation of events and speculating about alternative explanations of what might be going on, admit to yourself that his explanation just could be the correct one and as such should be considered seriously and investigated further.

Do not worry that you might be 'colluding' with the delusion – concerned interest and suspended disbelief will not strengthen the patient's conviction in his belief but it will provide a solid platform from which to challenge it.

WORKING WITH PARANOID PATIENTS

Trainee therapists are often concerned that if they appear to question the patient's paranoid beliefs then the patient will interpret this as a sign that they are part of the persecutory conspiracy and that they will become incorporated into his delusional system. If this does happen then clearly your ability to function as a CBT therapist is substantially reduced. Indeed, in such cases your therapeutic goal would probably be no more ambitious than to re-establish trust, to modify your patient's paranoid beliefs about yourself and then perhaps to use this modification as a starting point for a CBT programme. However, in practice you can nearly always avoid being drawn into the patient's paranoid system by ensuring that you have established a good trusting relationship with him before you express any doubts about his version of events or start to attempt belief modification, and by taking care to proceed very slowly and to be on constant alert to back off if necessary.

It is important to remember in this context that it is not the questions themselves that are likely to make your patient feel threatened so much as the way in which you ask them and how you react to his answers. It is normal practice in human society to ask questions because you want to know the answer and therefore it is also normal practice in human society to accept the answer you get. For example, I would not ask a colleague when the canteen was open if I already had this information, and if he told me it opened at 12 o'clock, he would not expect me to say he was wrong and that actually it opened at 12.30. Therefore, if you ask your patient a question and then imply that you do not believe his answer, it is not surprising if he takes offence. As we have already seen, the difficulty for you as therapist is that even if your words are neutral you can inadvertently convey your own opinions by the tone of your voice, the phraseology you use and even by the words you stress as you speak them. Practice in this way of working will increase your sensitivity to the covert message you imply by the way you say things to your patient but if you are genuinely able to take the position of suspending your disbelief about what he tells you then this is probably the best way of ensuring that you do not inadvertently signal rejection of his view of things or appear to be attempting to impose your own.

When interacting with a paranoid patient, do not rely on subtle social cues to indicate that you are non-threatening. There is research evidence to suggest that some people with schizophrenia may fail to detect the more subtle social cues in interpersonal interaction, and if your patient is already feeling threatened then it may require correspondingly more obvious or powerful indications from you that you are not the source of this threat. Smiling is a universal and powerful way of signalling friendly intent, so it may be appropriate to reassure your patient by smiling frequently. Or it may be appropriate to state explicitly what normally you would only imply, for example by telling the patient in so many words that you like and respect him and do not want any harm to come to him. It is perhaps surprising how often patients can be reassured of your good intent by using these basic social strategies.

SOME COMMONLY ENCOUNTERED PROBLEMS WITH THERAPY SESSIONS: SOME PRACTICAL SOLUTIONS

The patient is unco-operative with treatment of any kind

Patients admitted under a Section of the Mental Health Act may have no insight into their illness and therefore see all the staff as agents of a plot to keep them in hospital and force them to take unwanted medication. In these cases it may be appropriate for the therapist to distance himself from the ward team (e.g. 'I didn't know about your Section or have anything to do with it' or 'I don't have anything to do with medication and I'm afraid I can't influence your doctor about that one way or the other') in order to build up rapport. Rapport is built by showing interest and concern. In the most sensitive cases you have to be particularly careful not to express any doubts about what the patient tells you, if necessary explaining that you are powerless to do anything about the problem he describes. If there are any practical or any other issues that you can help with, then you should do so, even if it is not strictly in your job description as a therapist. For example, recently I have arranged for DSS benefits to be paid to one patient and for a minister to attend the ward to give communion to another. As far as possible, you should do these things yourself rather than delegating them elsewhere, first because then you can be sure they will be done promptly but, perhaps more importantly, because your own efforts will demonstrate your good will and genuine wish to help your patient.

The patient sees no reason to attend

One of the major challenges when working with people with schizo-phrenia is to get them interested and engaged in the therapy. Negative symptoms may impair your patient's motivation to co-operate and for some people with schizophrenia the social interaction involved in one-to-one therapy may not be as rewarding as it is for most people. Added to this, if your patient denies having any symptoms that need treating, there is the difficulty of explaining what your therapy might have to offer him.

The patient's failure to use cognitive techniques and practical coping strategies to counter his delusions and hallucinations, what is sometimes described as 'lack of motivation', can be frustrating for the therapist but it should not surprise us since it follows almost inevitably from the belief that the delusion is true. The unreasonableness of expecting people to detect and challenge their delusional beliefs can be demonstrated using our own beliefs and behaviour. For example, how often today have you questioned in your own mind if you are really the person you believe yourself to be, if you really are a mental health worker, etc.? How often has it occurred to you that you might not really be reading this book, that it might be an elaborate hallucination? I assume that you have done none of these things, and indeed it would be highly dysfunctional for you in everyday life if you were to constantly check what you 'know' to be the truth. The problem is that people with schizophrenia also 'know' that their delusions or hallucinations are true and therefore it does not occur to them to check these out either. In case you are tempted to argue that your certainties are based on objective reality and therefore are essentially different from the certainties based on delusional beliefs and psychotic experiences, I would ask you how often you have queried your certainty whilst you have been in the midst of a dream. Dreams can present us with bizarre situations and impossible sequences of events and yet whilst we are dreaming them we do not question their reality; we accept completely what seems to us, at the time, to be self-evidently real, or we just do not think about it one way or the other. I would suggest that until we routinely doubt and question what we know to be true in our everyday lives, and until we are able to detect every time we are dreaming and successfully challenge our experiences of 'reality' whilst we are dreaming, we are not in a position to feel frustrated or critical in any way of a patient who is unable to see that his delusional beliefs might not be true or who fails to use the helpful coping strategies that we have suggested to him. Indeed, I am constantly both humbled and impressed by the people who are able to challenge their certainties and who are able to use their rational, reasoning abilities to counter the very persuasive feelings of reality that accompany their experiences.

Without the usual motivation for therapy, i.e. the hope that the sessions will make him feel better, you have to provide the patient with other motivation. Taking time to talk to the patient about what he likes to talk about and offering tea/coffee and biscuits are two easy ways of making the session pleasant.

If the patient's condition fluctuates then you should be prepared to be flexible about appointments. Do not insist that your patient comes for his session if he is unwilling; for example, if he feels unwell it is better to express concern that he seems not to be feeling so good today, hope that he will soon feel better and then give him another appointment. If it is the distance or strangeness of your office that is putting the patient off, then try to see your patient in his own home territory (providing it is safe for you to do so) or on the ward if he is an inpatient. Once you have built up your relationship and he is more positive about the sessions, then you are in a better position to suggest appointments in your office.

Some people with schizophrenia do not find social contact rewarding in the way that most people do and a few find close or one-to-one contacts positively aversive. If your patient is reluctant to attend therapy sessions because he finds close social interactions uncomfortable or unpleasant, you should keep the sessions short and consider seeing him less frequently. Eye contact may be perceived as threatening rather than showing interest, so if your patient is reluctant to catch your eye you should take the hint and drop yours, only occasionally flicking to see if he wants to make eye contact. Also, pay attention to how your chairs are positioned within the room. Putting your chairs at a 90° angle will effectively distance you from your patient and will naturally avoid eye contact unless this is actively sought. Depending on the size of your room, it may also be feasible to increase the distance between your chairs. On one occasion I had sessions with a patient in a large room with our chairs separated by at least 15 feet; this felt really quite uncomfortable to me but with this arrangement he was able to stay for periods of up to half an hour whereas previously I had been unable to persuade him to sit down with me in a one-to-one situation.

Forgetfulness

A patient may be disorganised or just forget to attend sessions. Keeping to regular appointment times may help him to remember or he may agree to your giving him a reminder, for example by ringing him or a member of staff at his hostel or ward prior to the arranged session. In some cases, it may be simpler and more effective to arrange to go to him rather than vice versa, for example if he rarely leaves his hostel or ward.

Needless to say, it is not appropriate to adopt the approach taken in some therapies that the therapist's responsibility for meeting with the patient ends when he has offered the appointment that the patient must make a positive commitment to therapy by attending the appointment. When working with people with schizophrenia, you have to be more active in pursuing appointments; poor motivation and organisation are an integral part of schizophrenia and so arrangements for therapy sessions have to take this into account.

Thought disorder and idiosyncratic language

If the patient is thought disordered you may still be able to follow the general themes of what he is saying and work therapeutically with these. However, communication difficulties do mean that therapy takes longer, and the thought disorder can be frustrating for the therapist as the patient always seems to slide off the point just as you are about to ask the all important question. CBT cannot be used while the thought disorder is so severe that you are unable to follow what the patient is saying.

Do not assume that your patient is using terms or language in exactly the same way that you would. If you do not recognise a word or if your patient seems to be using a word in a way that does not quite make sense to you, then ask questions to clarify what he means.

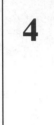

4

CBT with delusions and hallucinations: the course of therapy

INTRODUCTION

The major components of the cognitive behavioural treatment of delusions and hallucinations are described in Chapters 5–14. The long-term strategies for delusions and hallucinations comprise the cognitive strategies that the patient has found to be the most useful during the course of therapy, together with other more practical coping strategies and relapse prevention work: these are covered in Chapter 15.

It is recommended that you refer to the overall summary given in Appendix 2 as you read through these chapters, to enable you to put the various components and techniques described into the context of the full range of CBT strategies that is available.

FLEXIBILITY OF TREATMENT

The treatment programme for a particular patient could involve one or more of the major components and could use some or all of the possible strategies within those components.

Whilst the stages of therapy described in the next ten chapters are given in an order that would be appropriate for therapy, this order should not be considered a fixed one. The various strategies of treatment are to some extent interdependent and develop alongside one another so with any one patient you could be working with different strands at the same time, moving from one strand to another and back again in order to pursue and strengthen a particular line of approach. Thus, a typical programme with delusions would be to work to increase the patient's insight at the same time as starting the work to modify the delusional beliefs themselves, but full insight might not be reached until the delusional beliefs were successfully modified. Similarly, a typical programme with hallucinations would be to work with the content of the hallucination and the belief about its origin and significance at the same time as working to improve the patient's insight about his illness. With any one patient you might also be flexible in moving from one delusion to another or from delusion to hallucination, working on whichever aspect of each delusion and hallucination seems to be the most acceptable and beneficial for the patient at that time.

The skill of being able to move flexibly from one aspect of the work to another is an important one for the therapist to acquire, though in practice it is difficult to teach and is best gained through experience. In CBT with schizophrenia, there is no set way of doing things and usually no 'correct' way with any one patient. The only real guide as to the best approach to adopt for your individual patient is your sensitivity to his reaction as the different strategies are tried, so you need to be constantly on the alert to detect any resistance or adverse reaction from your patient. Providing you have set the goals of therapy, have good reasons for pursuing the approach you are using and are prepared to move slowly, backing off if necessary, you are unlikely to go wrong; the worst that will happen is that you will take longer to achieve the modification than is strictly necessary. Remember, providing you do not lose your patient's good will and co-operation, you can always come back to an unsuccessful strategy at some time in the future, when different circumstances and levels of insight may make it more acceptable and beneficial.

The one major proviso to this flexibility of approach is that **you must not start modifying a delusion unless and until you have ascertained that the new belief, when acquired, will be more acceptable and more functional for the patient than his old delusional belief.** For example, the goal might be to modify a patient's belief that his voices came from the devil to a belief that they were a symptom of schizophrenia. If he is horrified at the idea of having schizophrenia then you would have to make this acceptable to him **before** tackling his delusional explanation.

CBT AS AN ADJUNCTIVE TREATMENT TO MEDICATION

In our practice within the Specialist Services Unit we always use CBT as an adjunctive treatment to medication (i.e. given in addition to medication). Although nearly all the people admitted to our wards are deemed to be 'medication resistant', this does not mean that medication has no effect on them at all but rather that despite medication, often in high dosages, there are still substantial, uncontrolled symptoms of the illness that require the person to be hospitalised. With such severe levels of psychosis it would clearly be inappropriate to take them off medication or attempt to treat their symptoms with CBT alone. Without medication their psychotic experiences would be so overwhelming that any attempts to hold them with psychological techniques would be fruitless and even to consider otherwise is to fail to understand the profundity of their psychotic experiences. For people admitted to our unit, the standard practice is for their medication to be adjusted in order to achieve the best possible control of their symptoms by biochemical means and then CBT is used to counter and treat their often substantial residual symptoms.

Although we do not recommend CBT as an alternative to medication, clinical experience from our unit does suggest that once CBT has been established there may be less need for prn medication, and it may be that future studies will show that medication levels during the non-acute phases of the illness can be reduced where CBT is successful in dealing with the minor fluctuations in symptoms. Being able to reduce medication levels would be particularly beneficial for people who are experiencing significant side effects or where the side effects lead to non-compliance. It may be that some people with milder forms of the illness will be able to control their symptoms with CBT alone and they may choose to use CBT in preference to medication, but we have had very little experience with this level of illness in our unit. What we do know is that CBT cannot prevent recurrence of the delusional mood and experiences when the psychosis is active; CBT can only prevent the symptoms escalating and help to control dysfunctional behaviour whereas medication can actually prevent the delusional mood at source. Furthermore, even where CBT is effective, it may require considerable effort from the person concerned to apply it. Therefore, unless the medication is not effective or unless the unpleasant side effects of the medication outweigh its advantages, we would expect even mildly affected people to prefer to control their symptoms with medication rather than with CBT on its own.

WHO IS SUITABLE FOR CBT?

At the present time, we cannot tell with any degree of certainty who will benefit from CBT and who will not, or how long treatment might take to be effective. Clinical experience suggests that CBT will be more difficult and/or take longer the greater the patient's conviction in his delusions and the greater his involvement in them, but as some patients with firmly held delusions and hallucinations have responded positively to treatment I would not want to use this as a guide for excluding patients. I have a simple rule of thumb: if the patient is prepared to sit down with me then I will have a go to see if there is anything at all that I can do using CBT strategies. If you take such an all-inclusive approach there are bound to be patients for whom you will apparently be able to do nothing, but even in these cases your time will not have been wasted as it is likely that your patient will benefit in other ways from the therapeutic relationship. I have another simple rule of thumb: if the patient continues to want to see me then he must be getting something beneficial out of the sessions even if it is not the gains from CBT that I had been hoping for.

WHEN TO DELIVER TREATMENT

We noted in Chapter 2 the theoretical reasons why the most effective time to conduct CBT would be when the patient was at his least psychotic. Therefore, for patients who are severely ill and who are being treated in longer-stay units, it makes sense to wait until an appropriate medication regime has been established before starting CBT. Unfortunately, the present state of the NHS means that, especially in admissions wards, patients tend to be discharged as soon as there is a favourable response to medication and so usually it is necessary to start CBT before the optimal biological state has been achieved. Once the patient is living in the community then medication compliance becomes more problematic and so here also the therapist may have no choice but to deliver the CBT whilst the psychosis is only poorly controlled. So, whilst bearing the theoretical ideal in mind, in practice you should probably take the oppor- tunity to see the patient for CBT whenever and wherever it arises.

THE NUMBER AND SPACING OF THERAPY SESSIONS

It is likely that you will need to spend a lot of time just building up rapport and trust between you and your patient. This can be particularly time consuming if your patient lacks insight and denies having any illness or symptoms that could be treated. Where there is no insight and the patient is resentful about being in hospital, perhaps under a Section, it may take weeks or even months to build up sufficient rapport to be able to start tackling the delusions or hallucinations. With one patient who adamantly denied that she had a mental illness and would walk off in an angry huff if anyone suggested she had, I kept up contact for over a year before being able to talk about schizophrenia in even the most general of terms. In such cases (fortunately rare in this extreme) it may be better to use informal meetings with the patient to establish rapport, for example in a group or stopping to chat for five minutes when you meet on the ward, rather than asking the patient to visit you for longer, formal sessions.

There is no correct length for a CBT session. Normally we allocate one hour for each therapy session but it can be shorter, for example if the patient finds the one-to-one social situation difficult or if he is easily distracted by thoughts of other things he has to do. Even when well into therapy, it is not uncommon for much of the session to be composed of general conversation or discussing other concerns of the patient, with less than half of the session being used to push the cognitive programme along. Some patients may not feel confident or secure enough to talk about their psychotic experiences until they have spent some time talking about more neutral things, whereas other patients may be keen to talk about their concerns early on in the session but then need time to 'wind down' with more relaxing or reassuring conversation. For some patients with thought disorder, it is noticeable that they can engage in a meaningful dialogue for 20 minutes or so before their thoughts become too muddled, so in these cases you would aim to cover the CBT work in the early part of the session and be prepared just to listen to your patient in the latter part. When the psychosis is in relapse it may not be possible to progress the CBT at all, but nevertheless the session is not wasted if it can be used to support and help the patient through this difficult period.

Normally we see patients for therapy once a week, not least because this helps everyone to remember when the appointment is for, but there is no correct frequency. It may be appropriate to see some patients more often, for example if they will be in hospital for only a short while, or less often, for example if they find the sessions difficult and are only coming along to be obliging rather than because they positively want to. From our limited experience with frequent sessions, we would recommend that you do not have more than two or three active CBT sessions in each week because more frequent sessions can make even the most willing patient feel pressurised; furthermore, patients seem to need breathing space to consolidate what has been covered in the previous session. This is not to say that you should not meet your patient more frequently, only that you should not be attempting to cover new ground each time.

INFORMALITY OF APPROACH

When working with non-psychotic disorders, it is usual to start each session by recapping what was done the previous session, discussing the results of the homework assignment and then planning together what work you will cover in the present session. However, we have already noted that as a general rule we cannot discuss delusions and hallucinations in the same direct way that we would use for non-psychotic disorders and so neither can we adopt such a formal approach to the discussion of treatment. Although at the end of the previous session you will probably have noted useful issues to pursue in the next session, it is unlikely that you will be able to have a detailed discussion with your patient about the structure of each session and you should be prepared to deviate from your plan should your patient wish to pursue another line.

Although the approach to treatment sessions with people with schizophrenia is typically much more flexible, informal and unstructured than CBT with non-psychotic disorders, this does not mean that the therapist can be unstructured or imprecise in his thinking. Indeed, in many ways the informality of the treatment session itself means that the therapist must be all the more structured and focused about the plan of treatment.

THE USE OF GROUPS

Nearly all the CBT work we do with our patients is on an individual, one-to-one basis. We have tried using groups, both informal, large groups and smaller, more directed groups, but have found they provide very limited opportunities for progressing CBT. The main problem with our particular patient group is that people are at such different levels of insight that it is impossible to sustain a level of acceptance or challenge that is appropriate for all the members. However, groups can serve two useful purposes, so if they are convenient to organise (as, for example, on an inpatient unit) then you should consider setting one up. First, they can provide a useful forum for some of the destigmatising and insight promotion work (see Chapter 7). Second, meeting patients in a group is a good and time-efficient way of building up rapport and trust before you start treatment. As part of the group, individual patients are not the focus of attention as they would be in a one-to-one session and new patients have the opportunity to see that the therapist is trusted and respected by the other patients.

When patients have better insight then group work may be an appropriate and supportive way of providing therapy. This can be particularly useful for discussing coping strategies, for example, the different ways that group members have found of coping with voices.

HOMEWORK ASSIGNMENTS

Although setting the patient work to do in between sessions is a normal part of CBT with non-psychotic disorders, in our experience people with schizophrenia are not good at completing written homework assignments, so progress tends to be restricted to the therapy sessions unless other staff are trained to continue the work in between sessions. Certainly, in our group of severely ill people, very few have been able to undertake any formal homework involving written records, though many more are able to carry out practical tasks and then report back about them from memory. It may well be, however, that less severely ill patients would be able to participate in more ambitious homework exercises, so it is worth discussing this with your individual patient. For those who are unable to do the more complex homework tasks, the implication is that work between sessions must be kept simple and may need to be repeated over several weeks.

WARNINGS FOR THERAPISTS – IT'S EASIER SAID THAN DONE

Like many worthwhile things in life, CBT in schizophrenia is easier to describe in principle than it is to achieve in practice. It is important, therefore, that as a therapist you do not become discouraged by slow or erratic progress, or indeed by no progress at all. At the time of writing, the only patients who receive CBT are those who have significant and distressing psychotic symptoms despite being on medication, so the patients you will be working with are likely to be amongst the most severely ill. Bearing this in mind, you can see that any improvement at all resulting from your interventions must be considered a real and worthwhile achievement.

The therapist may have unrealistic expectations of success

For a therapist working in this field, it is dysfunctional to have underlying beliefs that have high expectations of success, such as 'I ought to be able to help my patients' or 'I ought to be able to help most of my patients most of the time' or 'If I were better at therapy I would be able to get positive results with this patient', etc.

More functional and realistic underlying beliefs in this context might be 'With such a difficult illness to treat, any progress I can make will be a very positive success', 'It's better to go slowly, even if no progress is made, than to try to push ahead too quickly and risk making the patient worse', 'I know that not everyone with schizophrenia will respond to a CBT approach but since I don't know who will respond and who won't, I can give it a try' and 'Even if I make no progress in modifying the delusions and hallucinations, the patient is likely to benefit at another level from our relationship and the interest and special regard that I have for him, so I will not have wasted the time'.

Progress may be erratic

Because of fluctuations in the underlying psychosis, progress made in one session may appear to be completely lost by the next. If this happens you should proceed cautiously as this may not be a good time to try to push the therapy forwards, but it may be helpful to remember that it will be quicker to regain ground that you have already covered than it was to cover it for the first time.

Conviction in a belief may fall gradually as the challenging work continues but not infrequently the therapist feels as if no progress is being made at all, only to find that the belief change, when it does occur, occurs quite suddenly, often between sessions. So do not be discouraged or deterred from continuing with therapy if all your best efforts seem to be getting nowhere. The modification you are working towards could appear quite suddenly.

The beneficial effects of therapy may not be recognised by the patient

One effect to be aware of is that after successful modification some patients may dismiss their previously held delusional beliefs as if they had been of no significance for them. This can be disconcerting for the therapist, not least if it causes you to wonder if all the time you spent with the patient had really been necessary. I well recall with one of my early cases reporting to our ward team how pleased I was that we had been able to modify the patient's very distressing belief that she would be doomed to eternal damnation. On interview the patient certainly looked cheerful and agreed that she was not damned, a gratifying moment for me, but then went on to add that she did not think she could ever have really believed such a thing possible! Disconcerting as these denials or minimising of the previously held delusional beliefs may be for the therapist, from the cases we have seen we are now confident that this is a sign of a profound and secure belief change and as such should be welcomed. It is as if, looking back with the hindsight of the new firmly held belief, the patient cannot credit that he could ever have believed differently. It may also be a reassuring sign that you have done your work so slowly and thoroughly that the patient is able to attribute his new understanding to his own efforts rather than to your interventions.

Better safe than sorry

Provided that you are sensitive to your patient's reactions and allow therapy to progress at his rate, which may be zero, rather than trying to push on to obtain results, then the cognitive therapy approach to delusions and hallucinations is a safe one to practise. The guiding principle to use in this approach with this client group is not to press on with a particular strategy if you have any doubts about your patient's response. If anything of potential significance comes up during therapy that you are not sure how to use, it is better to go away and think about it in between sessions rather than pushing on straight away. You might find it helpful to discuss the case with a colleague or to seek advice from a more experienced therapist. If none of these options is available you should continue to meet with your patient for general supportive work until you get some indications from that as to possible ways to continue.

Setting appropriate goals for the modification of delusions and hallucinations

5

ETHICAL CONSIDERATIONS

In general clinical practice the patient comes to the therapist to request help in changing a particular aspect of his life, be it behavioural, emotional or cognitive, and it is the patient who is ultimately responsible for setting the goals of his therapy. But since a cardinal feature of delusions is lack of insight about the nature and accuracy of those beliefs, deluded patients are necessarily not able to be objective or to request help for their symptoms in this way. We have already seen that where there is lack of insight you cannot talk to the patient about his delusions and hallucinations in those terms or discuss possible 'treatment' for his 'symptoms', so in these cases you have no choice but to take the lead in making the initial decision to attempt to modify the delusions or hallucinations without first discussing with the patient the treatment you would like to offer him. In these circumstances you must be particularly careful not to infringe the patient's right of choice for treatment.

Goal setting for CBT is governed by the overall principle that no-one has the right to interfere with another's belief system unless there is good reason to do so. In particular, the fact that a belief or experience may be considered by others to be a 'symptom' of an illness is not of itself sufficient reason to attempt modification. The following guidelines are recommended for consideration before starting treatment:

1. CBT may be started if the patient understands and requests it or, having had the treatment explained to him, agrees to it. (This is the standard CBT position.)
2. CBT for a delusion or hallucination may be started without the patient's expressed consent if this delusion or hallucination is causing

distress to the patient and if there is reason to believe that modification would reduce that distress.

Caution: Because a delusion or hallucination causes distress to the patient, it does not necessarily mean that he would want it modified or removed; there may be secondary gains which are not always immediately apparent to the therapist and that may be intricately bound up with the psychotic experience itself. Religious delusions and delusions about special relationships are particularly likely to fall into this latter class. For example, one of our patients was distressed by the invasion of the spirit world into his mind but he did not want this to stop because it was a significant religious experience for him. Another patient would become quite distressed by the critical messages sent over the airwaves by her parents, but although these messages were always unpleasant she did not want to lose this only remaining contact with her parents.

Although you may not be able to discuss the issue of modification directly with your patient, it is incumbent on you to find out by indirect questioning whether the modification you are considering would be an outcome welcomed by him. Some questions that I have found helpful in deciding whether or not the patient would want his beliefs or voices to be changed include:

'What don't you like about ... or hearing ...?' 'Are there any good aspects of... or hearing...?'

'What was it like before you realised ... or heard...?' 'Overall, was it better or worse, were you happier or less happy than you are now?'

'Suppose you woke up one morning and found it had all been a dream/nightmare, would you be relieved? Is there anything at all you might miss?' (If the patient is particularly sensitive about being believed it may be necessary after posing this question to reassure the patient that this is only a hypothetical question to find out what it must be like to be in the patient's situation, that you are not actually suggesting that he *could* wake up and find it had all been a mistake or dream.)

'Suppose the doctors were right and ... is not really..., that you think that way because of an illness, would that be good news for you or would that be worse than..., knowing that...?' (Putting this line of question does imply that the patient's explanation of events could be mistaken and so it should only be used where this would not threaten rapport or trust for future CBT.)

3. It is not uncommon for delusional beliefs to have both positive and negative consequences for the patient. In these cases it is appropriate to consider whether the gain to the patient from holding to the belief

could be got from elsewhere and if so, to work with the patient to establish this new source of 'gain' before attempting modification. For example, a patient who believed he was a senior member of the secret service gained a great sense of self-esteem and purpose from the belief, but the disadvantage for him was that he would come into conflict with the law when he shoplifted electronics equipment that he needed for his work for the government. Inconvenient as this latter behaviour was, it was decided not to attempt modification of the core belief unless and until the sense of self-esteem it gave could be provided from elsewhere. In such cases, whether or not you proceed with the modification and/or what goals you set may depend on how successful you have been in substituting the beneficial parts of the delusion so that the delusion is no longer needed to supply them.

4. If a delusion or hallucination is causing distress to others rather than to the patient himself it may be ethical to start CBT without the patient's expressed consent providing there would be no loss for the patient by such a modification and some expected secondary gain for him. For example, when one of our patients became unwell she would believe that another patient was her 'true biological father', an idea that she found intriguing rather than distressing but that her father found very upsetting. In this case modifying her belief caused her no loss but it had direct benefit for her father and, in the long run, benefit for her since her recognition of him as 'father' helped to reinforce his frequent visits and care.

   Preventing behaviour that distresses others normally does have some positive gain for the patient, for example by avoiding court procedures or enforced hospitalisation, improving relationships within the home and ensuring greater support from carers, etc. Therefore, the principal consideration before modifying a delusion in a way that will directly benefit others rather than the patient is whether or not that modification would have any actual negative effects for the patient, and if so, whether that would outweigh the positive gains.

5. If at any time during therapy it becomes apparent that there are some secondary gains from the symptoms that were not previously detected or if the patient appears not to want to lose his delusional beliefs or hallucinations, then therapy should be suspended whilst the situation is reviewed. Since the treatment will only have been started in the first place because there appeared to be some obvious gains for the patient in modifying his beliefs or hallucinations, it may be appropriate to set new goals for treatment, for example, a partial rather than total modification (see later section in this chapter). Alternatively, if there is a secondary gain that would be lost if the delusion were modified, then it would be appropriate to attempt to supply this 'gain' from

elsewhere before progressing with the modification (see point 3, above).

6. Grandiose delusions should be approached with great caution. It is probable that a grandiose delusion will not be distressing to the patient, in which case the primary reason for attempting to modify it, namely to alleviate the patient's distress, will not be there. Modification should only be attempted if the potential benefits of doing so clearly outweigh the possible disadvantages. The fact that a belief is delusional is never sufficient reason on its own for imposing treatment. Grandiose delusions often serve a very positive function for the patient of maintaining or boosting his self-esteem. Therefore, if there are clear benefits to be gained from modifying a grandiose delusion then you must seek to determine what the potential effects on self-esteem of removing the grandiose delusion will be and work on building up that self-esteem before modification is attempted. In many cases of grandiose delusion it is appropriate to go for a partial rather than total modification (see below) which allows those parts of the delusion that are important for self-esteem to be retained. Total modification of the grandiose delusion would normally be attempted only where a partial modification is not possible or would not be sufficient to produce the required positive effects, for example in the case of the patient who believed he had supernatural powers that would allow him to emerge unscathed if he threw himself in front of a bus.

PRACTICAL CONSIDERATIONS

A direct or insensitive challenge to a strongly held belief may actually strengthen conviction in that belief, so where a number of delusional beliefs are held, ideally you would start with the weakest belief first and modify that before moving on to the more strongly held beliefs. The advantages of starting with the weaker beliefs are fourfold. First, they are more likely to shift and to shift quickly, so the patient can feel some benefits from the therapy quite early on in the course of treatment. Second, using the CBT techniques with a weaker belief will enable the patient to learn and to get practice with those techniques in a situation where he is unlikely to experience any setbacks or resistance. Third, successful modification will provide the patient with evidence that believing something to be true does not necessarily guarantee that it is true. Furthermore, once the patient has discovered that he is capable of holding inaccurate beliefs he may be more prepared to consider that some of his more strongly held beliefs could also be inaccurate. Last but not least, starting with the weaker beliefs will be easier for the therapist. With weakly held beliefs there is less risk of adverse reaction if you make a wrong move and you will be able to get to know your patient better and build up trust before tackling the stronger beliefs.

Although there are good theoretical reasons for attempting to modify weaker delusional beliefs before stronger, in practice you will often have to temper this with considerations of what the patient deems important and would like to have tackled first. If your patient is distressed about some major interest, it may come across as lack of understanding or concern if you concentrate on some minor, unimportant aspect of his life, and as a consequence he may drop out of therapy before you can get onto the more significant delusional beliefs.

WHAT SHOULD THE PATIENT END UP BELIEVING?

Setting the goals for modification of delusional beliefs is not just a question of deciding what the patient will stop believing; of equal importance is deciding what the patient will believe instead. We have already seen in Chapter 1 how our brains seek to understand and make sense of what is going on around us and the crucial importance that beliefs have in enabling us to do this. It is not surprising that if a patient comes to the point of rejecting a previously held delusional belief, he will necessarily form another belief to take its place in order to explain the events and experiences that were previously explained by the delusional belief. So, when seeking to modify a delusion, you must take care to use the appropriate strategies not only to disprove the delusion but also to shape up the new belief that will supersede it. If you fail to do this you may find that the delusional belief is merely replaced by another delusional belief, and this new delusion may be even more disruptive and harder to modify than the original one – definitely *not* a successful outcome for your intervention!

TOTAL AND PARTIAL MODIFICATION

The aim of CBT with schizophrenia is not to get rid of a delusion just because it is a 'symptom' of the illness, it is not to modify a delusion just so that the belief is nearer to the 'truth' and it is not to make the delusional belief more socially acceptable or politically correct. The aim of CBT with delusions is to reduce the distress caused by those delusions. This being so, it is not always necessary to modify the core delusional belief to achieve therapeutic gain; indeed, in some cases modifying the core delusional belief might actually cause the patient unhappiness. Therefore, in some cases, the best overall therapeutic gain may be achieved by modifying only those parts of the delusional system that cause problems for the patient.

The two types of modification to be considered when setting the goals for modification are total and partial.

Total modification

In a total modification the end result is the complete rejection of the previously held delusional belief and its replacement by some other, incompatible belief. For example, a total modification for the patient who believed he was Hitler reincarnated might be 'I am not a reincarnation of Hitler and never have been: I thought I was Hitler because I was getting strange feelings about not being myself and having done something terrible in the past, but these feelings were due to my brain not working properly because of the illness I had'.

Partial modification within the delusional system

In a partial modification only those parts of the delusional system causing problems for the patient are targeted for modification, and the goal of modification must be compatible with the parts of the delusional system that are left intact. In some cases partial modification may be the modification of choice, but in other cases it may be the only one achievable when attempts at a total modification have failed.

If a delusional belief affords the patient some secondary gain that cannot be replaced from elsewhere then a partial modification is the modification of choice. For example, one of our patients believed he was the son of a royal prince. This caused problems at home because talking about this royal connection caused rows between him and his father. When asked what it would be like if he were not the son of royalty, the patient told us that this would be terrible (for reasons connected with other parts of his delusional system). So at least in the short term, a complete modification of this belief was deemed to be undesirable. The goal of partial modification in this case was for the patient to change his beliefs about the old man he lived with, to recognise that the old man did not know that the patient had royal blood but genuinely believed himself to be the patient's father. With this part of the belief system modified, the patient saw that it would be unkind to the elderly man to talk about his 'real' father at home and so he refrained from doing so. In this way damaging conflicts between the patient and his father were avoided but he retained the benefits of his belief about royal parentage.

Note: Focusing on what other people believe can be a particularly useful partial modification for grandiose delusions. Grandiose delusions often cause trouble not so much because of what the person believes about himself as what the patient believes other people believe about him. For example, believing himself to be a member of the royal family did not of itself cause any problems for one of our patients but the problems came when he expected other people to do things for him at the snap of his fingers. Modifying the patient's belief about what other people believe does not challenge the core delusional belief about what or who the patient is, but it does prevent the conflicts that can arise when other people are expected to behave as if they believe the same things. Modifications of what the patient believes about other people's beliefs can also be useful in other situations where it is not desirable or possible to modify the core delusional belief, and so this particular form of modification should always be borne in mind.

Where the partial modification is chosen in order to protect some aspect of the delusional system then you have to be careful that the new modified parts of the belief will not create a challenge to the parts you want to keep intact. This latter is most likely to occur if the new part of the belief is incompatible with the parts being left untouched or if the situations involved are so similar that the work done to modify the unwanted part generalises to the other part. For example, a patient was hearing the voices of God and other spirits, some supporting but others very unpleasant, critical and threatening. Partial modifications to change the beliefs about the unpleasant voices were considered; the goal of this modification would have been that the voice of God was genuine but that the other voices were inaccurate perceptions due to misinterpretations of his brain. However, the importance of hearing God was so great for this patient (when asked what it would be like if God no longer talked directly to him, the patient replied that it would be awful and that he would commit suicide) that it was too risky to challenge the authenticity of the other voices in case a successful challenge should trigger him to question the voice of God in the same way. Thus, in some cases even a partial modification is not safe to attempt, i.e. if there is a risk that this could threaten a core delusional belief that would be damaging to the patient to remove.

Although a total modification may be the goal of choice, you may be able to get positive therapeutic gain with a partial modification if total modification is not successful. For example, one of our patients had been referred to us from the courts after he had seized a policeman's walkie-talkie and smashed it to the ground. On a couple of occasions prior to this he had noticed that his eyesight and hearing were affected when he was near one of these sets in use, and as a result had developed the firmly held belief that some of the walkie-talkie sets used by traffic police are 'duff' and can affect his and other people's sight and hearing. According to his belief it was perfectly reasonable, and indeed even socially responsible, to approach a policeman using one of the 'duff' sets and ask him politely to switch it off – and to smash the offending instrument to the ground when the policeman did not respond as requested. This was perfectly reasonable behaviour because it was the only way to protect his and other people's senses. The problem for the patient was that if he smashed another walkie-talkie after discharge he would be returned to hospital or prison. Since there were no positive gains to this delusional belief about the walkie-talkies we attempted a complete modification, the goal of which was 'Walkie-talkies cannot affect anyone's sight or hearing, the odd experiences I had before were nothing to do with the walkie-talkie sets being used and could have been due to...'. But despite trying many different approaches we had no success. (I have noticed over the years that delusions based on people's sensory experiences are particularly difficult to modify, presumably because normally our senses are accurate and reliable sources of information and therefore to be trusted without question.) We discussed coping strategies to keep him away from the offending walkie-talkies but he did not feel these would be successful because he had a duty to protect other people's sight and hearing as well as his own. This discussion was helpful because it suggested that a partial modification could be effective in controlling the undesired behaviour, this modification being about the walkie-talkies' effects on other people's sight and hearing. As he did not have the same sensory evidence to back up his belief about the adverse effects of the radio waves on other people, we were able to successfully modify this belief so that he ended up by believing that only his sight and hearing could be affected. Having achieved this partial modification, we were then able to agree a set of coping strategies, such as removing himself from the 'duff' set as soon as he felt its adverse effects. Knowing that he had no responsibility for other people, that he only had to look after himself, swung the balance away from him smashing the sets to taking evasive action should he encounter a 'duff' set in operation in the future.

Deciding whether to go for a total or partial modification

Total modifications are the goal whenever there are no positive gains to the patient in holding his delusional belief, because total modifications are more secure than partial modifications against future relapse. This is because once the delusional idea has been rejected, the replacement belief can be slotted into and therefore supported by the patient's existing network of rational, non-delusional beliefs. If part of the delusional system is left intact there is always the potential that, being compatible with the delusional beliefs, the remaining section of the delusion will reactivate the parts that had been modified and overlaid. For example, in the case just mentioned, with only a partial modification there is still the possibility that some other people's sight and hearing might be affected by the walkie-talkies, so if he should notice people looking perplexed or moving away from the policeman when he gets the experience again, then he may conclude that perhaps these particular people are like him in being vulnerable to the radio waves and that therefore he should 'protect' them by smashing the 'duff' set.

The following questions may be helpful in deciding whether to go for a complete or partial goal.

1. Why is the delusional belief causing distress or having an adverse effect on the patient's life and how does it do this?
2. Are there any advantages for the patient in holding this belief? If not, consider the goal of total modification. It is good practice to speculate about the advantages and disadvantages of a patient's delusional beliefs but do not set goals on the basis of your speculation alone. Check them out first with your patient by asking neutral, non-challenging questions, such as 'What would it be like if...?' or 'Do you wish that ... wasn't so?' or 'Supposing...'. Then set the goals on the basis of his responses.
3. If there are some advantages to the patient in holding his belief, could they be replaced from elsewhere? If so, a total modification could still be considered if you are successful in replacing the source of positive gain by something else. If you are unable to do this, is it possible to achieve a partial modification that leaves the beneficial parts of the delusion intact?
4. If there are some advantages and some disadvantages in holding the belief, is it possible to do a partial modification? What bits of the delusional belief should stay intact? What are the goals for the parts being changed, i.e. what will the patient end up believing? Are these new beliefs compatible with the parts of the delusional system left intact or would the partial modification have unwanted knock-on effects on the parts of the system to be retained?
5. If a partial modification is not possible, does the overall gain from a total modification outweigh the losses or is it better for the patient that his whole system be left intact?
6. If a total modification has been unsuccessful, could a partial modification be therapeutically useful and achieved in practice?

Adapting the goal of treatment as treatment progresses

Although you should not start to modify a delusion until you have specified the end goal towards which you are working, and any intermediate goals that you may need to reach in between, you may need to change these goals during therapy. We have just considered that it may be necessary to change from a total to a partial modification goal if it turns out not to be possible in practice to achieve the total modification. Another situation that may arise is where your patient gives you some new information which suggests that the 'ideal' goal is not ideal after all. For example, it may emerge that there are previously unsuspected advantages to the patient in holding certain aspects of his belief or that the new goal is incompatible with some deeply held, non-psychotic belief. In these circumstances you should not hesitate to change the goal of treatment to a more appropriate one.

SETTING THE GOAL

Example from clinical practice

The patient described his situation as follows:

> In a previous reincarnation I was King Henry VIII. I vividly recall events from my life in those times and I recognise some of the people I lived with then who are alive now. Sometimes I get very angry when my subjects refuse to do as they're told. I do not expect people who were not members of my household to serve and wait on me, though they should treat me with respect once they know who I am. The hostel staff tell me I should do normal household chores like washing my clothes but a king should not do these things. I am a very important person and I have the right to punish my subjects if they fail to obey me. Yesterday I hit one of my servants who refused to give me a cigarette.

This was typical of grandiose delusions in that the problems arose not because of the patient's core belief that he was Henry VIII or even because he believed he recognised other people who had been alive with him at that time; the problems arose because of the associated beliefs that these people knew about their previous reincarnations and recognised him as their king but then failed to act accordingly.

A total modification, in which the new belief would have been that he had not been Henry VIII, could have had adverse effects on the patient if his self-esteem were in any way tied up with having been a powerful king. This possibility could have been checked out first by asking the patient in general how one incarnation affects another, what influence previous lives have on our present ones, etc. and then by asking him in particular how his present life would be different if he had been someone else (e.g. a servant) in previous times and how he or other people might feel about that. It is very likely that total modification, even if it could have been achieved in practice, would have had some significant adverse effects on this patient's self-esteem; at the very least it would have required him to accept that what he had been asserting for so long to so many people was only a delusion and furthermore that other people recognised it as such. In this type of situation, before going on to consider whether the gains achieved from a total modification would outweigh the negative effects, it is better to ask whether a partial modification could be as effective in controlling the problems associated with the delusional beliefs. In cases where there is some positive gain from holding the delusional belief, if a partial modification would be as effective as a total modification at solving the problems associated with the delusion then the partial modification is indicated as the goal of choice. Not only is a partial modification more likely to be achievable but it also respects the general principle that we do not have the right to interfere with other people's beliefs any more than is necessary to achieve their well-being.

In this particular case, the problems identified were around aggression and sometimes violent behaviour towards people who did not obey the patient's commands. The key to the solution to this problem lies in his behaviour towards people he does not believe were reincarnated with him in his earlier life; he accepts that they do not recognise him as Henry VIII and therefore he does not expect them to treat him as such. Therefore, if he could come to an understanding that people do not recognise him as Henry VIII, even if he is sure he recognises them as being with him at that time, then this should be sufficient to stop him behaving dictatorially and aggressively towards them.

The partial modifications that would be effective in this case target the following aspects of his beliefs:

1. that he can correctly identify people's previous incarnations (if he can make mistakes about who people had been in the past then it would be inappropriate to give orders to people who might not have been his servants previously);
2. that other people are aware of their previous incarnations (if they are not aware of who they were then they cannot realise their obligations);
3. that other people recognise the patient as Henry VIII (if they do not recognise him then they cannot respond to him as a king).

Any one of these partial modifications could be effective in controlling the patient's behaviour but ideally one would attempt to use all three in order to strengthen that control. In practice, the modification around his ability to correctly recognise people from their previous lives (modification 1) is likely to be difficult to achieve, because although the former is actually a misidentification, nevertheless it still involves 'recognition', a powerful subjective experience that can carry with it its own sense of absolute certainty. Since we can never be as sure about other people's experiences as we can about our own, it should be easier to modify the patient's beliefs about other people's awareness of their previous lives and about their recognition of the patient (modifications 2 and 3).

Although the patient's core belief about being Henry VIII reincarnated would be left intact by these partial modifications, it would be advisable to look at his beliefs about reincarnation to see whether any partial modification is required within this set of beliefs. A key aspect of his present belief about reincarnation that is causing problems is his belief that previous positions and relationships (e.g. between the king and his subjects) are also transferred to the new existence. This is contradictory to mainstream beliefs about reincarnation and as such modification might well be possible. If the patient were to believe instead that within any one reincarnation one's role and relationships with other people are determined by that incarnation and not previous ones, that the purpose of an incarnation is to experience what it is like living as that particular person in that particular role, then this would mean that it would be inappropriate for him to behave as a king in his present incarnation. This modification would help to strengthen the control on his behaviour whilst leaving intact his belief that reincarnation happens and that he was Henry VIII in a previous life.

The fact that the patient believes that people should treat him with respect once they realise who he was in previous times suggests that he is using this belief as a source of self-respect and esteem. This indicates that work to build up his self-esteem and confidence should be undertaken alongside the belief modification work.

Goal: Partial modification
Work on self-esteem

New beliefs: 1. Other people do not realise that they are reincarnations from previous times and do not recognise me as Henry VIII. Most people do not realise that reincarnation happens and so do not believe I was the king even when I tell them. Therefore, their failure to treat me as a king is due to ignorance rather than deliberate disrespect.
2. Roles and relationships that apply in one incarnation do not apply in another. Therefore, in this life I should not expect people to obey me as they did when I was the king.

THE ASSESSMENT PROCESS

It may take several sessions to gather the information necessary to make an assessment and plan therapy, but of course these are not wasted as they will be helping to build up the therapeutic relationship. Assessment is not a one-off process that is done as a prelude to therapy and then stops there. It continues throughout the course of therapy as new infor-

Table 5.1 Information required for goal setting and treatment planning

1. DELUSIONS
For each delusion:
 What is it?
 What evidence does the patient have to support it?
 Is the evidence a feeling, real fact, distorted fact or delusion?
 How firmly is it held?
 How distressing is it?
 How does it affect the patient's life?
 Are there any relevant (psychotic or non-psychotic) underlying beliefs?

2. HALLUCINATIONS
For each hallucination:
 What are the physiological characteristics of the voice?
 Where and who does it come from?
 How does the patient know the voice comes from a particular person/entity?
 What does the voice say (or what sort of thing does the voice say)?
 Does the voice tell the truth?
 What power/authority does the voice have?
 Can the voice or source of the voice harm the patient?
 Does the voice command the patient and, if so, how?
 Is the voice difficult to resist?
 What does or could happen if the patient resists?
 Does the patient have any evidence of the voice's power?
 How frequent is the voice?
 How distressing is the voice?
 How does it affect the patient's life?
 Are there any relevant (psychotic or non-psychotic) underlying beliefs affecting the content?

3. INSIGHT AND ATTITUDE TO SCHIZOPHRENIA
Does the patient acknowledge that he has an illness?
What is the patient's attitude to schizophrenia?
Does the patient relate the symptoms/experiences to his illness?
Would the patient be upset if his symptoms were attributed to 'illness'?

4. POTENTIAL PROBLEMS
e.g. Is the patient unwilling or unable to engage in therapy?

mation comes in and it may take many months before important issues emerge; for example, in one of our cases a key aspect of the problem, a hitherto unsuspected underlying belief, did not come to light until a follow-up session several years after therapy had begun. Therapy should be flexible and adaptable to incorporate the new information and updated assessment: thus treatment plans may change as therapy progresses and sometimes even the goals of treatment change.

6 | Prior to treatment: lessening the impact and distress caused by the delusions and hallucinations

INTRODUCTION

Before starting the formal CBT programme, it is appropriate to consider if there are any cognitive or practical ways of reducing the impact of the delusion or hallucination on the person's life and of lessening the distress that it can cause. This is not normally seen as part of the treatment itself but rather as a means of controlling the adverse effects of the symptoms whilst the CBT programme is being progressed. Whether or not it is possible to alleviate the distress prior to CBT treatment will depend on the content and nature of the delusion or hallucination concerned.

COGNITIVE STRATEGIES

Although in general we advocate the approach of allowing the possibility that the patient's belief just might be true and not delusional, of believing your patient until proven otherwise or at least suspending your disbelief, a major exception to this is when your patient is very distressed by his delusion or hallucination and does not want it to be true, and is reassured rather than irritated if other people say that they do not believe it to be true.

If the delusion could not be true in fact then it may be possible to lessen the distress it causes your patient by reassuring him that you do not believe as he does, explaining your reasons for not doing so. For example, one of our young female patients believed she had had 20 or more babies and killed them all. Although she was not persuaded by our arguments along the lines that she could not have had so many babies in that time, that someone would have noticed that she was pregnant, that she would have required medical treatment that would be recorded in her notes, etc., she did accept that if we were so sure she could not have done these things then perhaps there could just possibly be some doubt about it.

One of the advantages of giving reassurance at this early stage, always providing it is appropriate to do so, is that even though the arguments you present will probably not persuade your patient that his delusion is incorrect they may cast just a shadow of doubt in his mind, as with the patient above, and this may be enough to encourage him to think it is worthwhile exploring the issues further with you. Furthermore, even though your patient may not find your arguments persuasive he may find it mildly reassuring that everyone else does.

When searching for reasons why the delusion could not be true, a good starting point is to ask yourself why *you* think it could not happen. If you regard the patient's belief as delusional you must have good reasons for believing it to be improbable or impossible, and you may be able to harness some of these reasons to persuade your patient. It may well be that you have taken for granted that the delusional belief is not true and therefore do not have a comprehensive list of reasons to justify your assumption, in which case your task is to think the issue through and to come up with these reasons. When doing this exercise, do not forget to include the most obvious reasons, remembering that what seems obvious to you may not have occurred to your patient in connection with his delusion. It is good practice to think of as many reasons as possible why the delusion cannot be true because the reasons that you find totally convincing may not impress your patient and vice versa, i.e. something that you find less persuasive may just ring a bell with your patient and be the one thing that he finds reassuring (see example below).

If the delusion or hallucination is about something that is going to happen in the future then it may be possible to lessen the distress by showing that the feared something could not happen or, if it could happen, that it would not matter if it did.

Example from clinical practice

One of our patients believed that two particular nurses wanted to put him in a coffin and transport him to the crematorium where he would be cremated alive. We tried several lines of reason as to why he could not be put into a coffin on the ward, which was what he feared, including that he could scream and shout and fight back if either of the nurses tried to seize him, that other staff whom he did trust would come to protect him when they saw or heard what was happening, that it would not be possible for either of the nurses to purchase a coffin without incriminating records of their purchase being kept, to carry a coffin up the stairs into the ward without being seen or to hide anything as large as a coffin on the ward. He accepted these arguments but did not find any of them convincing.

Having been unable to persuade him that it would be impossible for the nurses to remove him from the ward in a coffin, we looked at the later stage of the feared event that dealt with the coffin being burnt in a crematorium. We thought it was highly unlikely that a body could be burnt without stringent checks that it was dead so we did some research to discover what those checks might be. We found that in order to be cremated a body has to be seen and certified as dead by at least four independent people (doctors and undertakers). Our patient accepted that since he would be alive in the coffin when the doctors and undertakers saw him there was no way they could make a mistake and think he was dead. He also accepted that these four independent people did not know him and therefore could have nothing against him and therefore would not want to be involved in his murder. He found this a persuasive line of argument and was able to use it to counter the distress caused by the delusional thoughts when they occurred.

Accepting that the security measures at the crematorium meant there was no possibility of his being burnt alive enabled our patient to effectively counter the delusional thoughts when they occurred, so then we turned our attention to modifying his belief that these members of staff *wanted* to do this to him. This latter was important for two reasons. First, it must be very unpleasant to think that anyone would want to kill you, especially in such an unpleasant way, even if you think they could not possibly carry out the act, so it was important to remove this unpleasant idea. Second, just showing that it would not be possible in practice for the nurses to have him cremated alive would be a much weaker and more vulnerable form of therapy than tackling the underlying belief. Doubts about the safety afforded by the independent signatures procedures could always creep in; for example, he might get the thought that the nurses had bribed the doctors to say that he was dead or that no-one might notice the extra coffin being slipped on to the incinerator slide or, persuaded that the nurses could not kill him by cremating him, he might have developed the delusion that they would try to poison him or kill him in some other way.

Deciding what level of reassurance to give

When deciding whether or not to come off the fence immediately with respect to your patient's delusions or hallucinations in favour of a definite reassurance that you do not believe them to be true, the deciding factor is not the level of disturbance or distress that the symptoms cause but how important it is to your patient that you give credence to his beliefs and interpretation of events. As we have already seen, some patients can be very distressed by their delusions or hallucinations and would much rather they were not true or did not happen, but nevertheless it is more important for them in the early stages of their relationship with the therapist that the therapist takes their position seriously and does not disagree with them or dismiss their version of what has been happening. Patients with firmly held delusional beliefs who have already spent some weeks or months in the mental health system can become extremely frustrated that no-one will accept their version of events or seems to understand exactly what has been going on. For them, having a therapist who will actually take their view seriously and not try to reassure them that they are wrong or worrying unnecessarily may well be far more important than hearing the same old thing as everyone else has said. For example, one of our patients believed she was inhabited by an ex-friend. This belief caused her great distress, not least because of what the ex-friend threatened to do to her. Nevertheless, she had become so angry and frustrated that people did not believe what she told them that any reassurance on my behalf that I, too, did not believe she was possessed would have led to instant breakdown of our emerging therapeutic relationship, because it would have indicated to her that I had also totally failed to grasp what was really going on.

As part of the assessment process, you will have asked your patient about his delusional beliefs and hallucinatory experiences in order to set appropriate goals for modification, so you will probably have a good indication from his responses to these questions what his attitude is towards being disbelieved. However, if you are not sure whether your patient would welcome your reassurance that you do not think his delusional belief is true, or whether he would take this as a sign that you had failed to understand him, then you can test the ground by starting with a tentative level of doubt (e.g. 'I don't think I can be as certain as you are that...') and getting more definite if your patient's response is favourable (e.g. 'That seems unlikely to me' or 'I'm pretty sure that can't be true'). You need to be sensitive not to push your level of certainty too far, however, because once you have firmly expressed your own views about the beliefs then you have intimated to your patient that you are attempting to prove to him that his delusion is not true rather than exploring with him whether or not it is true.

Caution: Strategies used to lessen the impact of a delusion often constitute an indirect challenge to the delusion and as such should be tried tentatively in the early stages of therapy; if there are any signs of resistance they should be discontinued. This line of approach can always be taken up again later in therapy when there is better insight.

PRACTICAL STRATEGIES

Delusions

In the midst of thinking about the more sophisticated treatment strategies that you could use, do not forget to consider whether any plain, simple, practical strategy could help to reduce the impact or distress caused by the delusion or hallucination. The following examples come from our clinical practice.

1. A patient was troubled by the voice of evil spirits when she woke in the night. These faded or disappeared in the light, so a simple strategy to relieve her distress was for her to sleep with the light on.
2. A patient's delusional beliefs were made worse when they were confirmed by people in TV programmes. A simple strategy to relieve the added distress was for him to avoid the TV lounge.
3. A patient was troubled by frightening delusional ideas when he woke up at night; he had similar ideas in the day but in a much milder form and less disturbing. A simple strategy was to readjust his bedtime and medication so that he did not wake in the middle of the night.

Hallucinations

Practical strategies have such an important role in helping to control hallucinations that they are considered separately, in Chapter 9.

The promotion of insight about delusions

7

THE REASON FOR PROMOTING INSIGHT

A core feature of a delusion is that the person holding it believes it to be true and therefore does not recognise it as a delusion; similarly, someone experiencing hallucinations will experience them as real events happening in the real world, not as some internally generated sensation. Even when patients acknowledge that they have a mental illness called schizophrenia it is not uncommon for them to deny that their beliefs or experiences are symptoms of that illness – it seems so self-evident that they are real that they cannot be doubted or recognised as being otherwise. It should not surprise us that this is so, given that delusional beliefs, once established, behave essentially like any other firmly held belief and that auditory hallucinations are actually 'heard' as coming from some external source. In practice, however, you will find that people often do seem to behave towards people with delusions and hallucinations as if 'somewhere deep down they must know, really, that it can't be true'. This latter is a good example of people being unable to leave their own beliefs behind when they try to put themselves in someone else's position, so that their own beliefs colour their imagination of how the other person must think and feel.

As we have already seen, when we considered the function of beliefs in Chapter 1, it is necessary for us to be able to make definite assumptions about the world in order to avoid being overwhelmed by the infinite complexity and variability that life presents, and in order for us to be confident in our assumptions, it is necessary for our brains to give us a sense of certainty in their correctness. The only disadvantage of this ability to confer this sense of certainty is that our brains can sometimes incorrectly attach it to ideas and experiences which are not, in fact, accurate reflections of objective reality. It is perhaps not surprising, though, that this incorrect attribution of certainty can be just as convincing for the person concerned.

This very 'real' quality that delusions and hallucinations have, the fact that they can appear to be so obviously 'true' to the person concerned, can have two very significant effects. First, it is probably the most important factor in determining the impact that the delusions and hallucinations have on the patient's life and the distress that these symptoms can cause: delusions and hallucinations are particularly disturbing and influential because of the reality that they signify. Second, whilst the patient believes his delusions and hallucinations to be a true reflection of what is going on in the world around him then the notion of 'illness' is necessarily irrelevant, as also is medication or any other form of treatment to alleviate the situation, including the use of many of the CBT strategies and coping behaviours.

Because of the impact that lack of insight about delusions and hallucinations can have for the patient, nearly all CBT programmes include some insight promotion work. The aim of this is to increase the patient's understanding of what is happening to him, to help him to understand his symptoms and to detect when his symptoms occur so that he can put appropriate coping strategies or treatments into effect.

In essence, the purpose of the insight promotion work is to enable the patient to take a detached, objective view of his subjective experiences, though as we have already seen, this may be very difficult to achieve in practice; subjective experiences, particularly those involving the senses, may be imbued with their own assurance of truth and reality which is just too convincing to be countered by arguments or apparently conflicting evidence. In some cases, therefore, it may not be possible for the patient to achieve full insight about his symptoms or illness even though this was included in the treatment goal of choice; in these cases, significant gains for the patient may still be possible if a partial insight can be achieved. Although full insight is usually the goal of choice there may be good reasons why this is considered undesirable for a particular patient, in which case you would consider whether partial insight, about just certain aspects of the illness or symptoms, was desirable.

PARTIAL INSIGHT

There are two broad classes of partial insight. First, there are the cases where the patient has made some movement away from believing that his experiences are entirely accurate indications of what is going on in the outside world, but where the cause of those experiences is still given as something other than illness or the brain not functioning properly. This sort of partial insight is usually more vulnerable to subsequent loss than full insight but nevertheless these partial, alternative explanations for the symptoms can function as a proxy for the full, illness explanation, and as such enable the patient to put into effect some appropriate coping strategies which would not have been possible when there was no insight at all. For example, one of our patients concluded that being in hospital helped to get rid of the evil spirits that invaded his mind because they could only get to him when he was not sleeping properly and when he was in hospital he was able to relax and take 'sleeping' tablets to help him sleep through the night. Another patient came to the understanding that when he went through periods of being up all night, chain smoking and drinking heavily, periods that he called 'high spirits', he was likely to have paranoid ideas. This was a therapeutic gain for the patient because it meant that when he was going through one of these 'high' periods, he would use cognitive strategies to test whether his ideas about having the phone tapped, etc. were accurate or whether they were caused by the 'high spirits'. Another of our patients came to the conclusion after some weeks of CBT that there was dust in the air that could make her 'imagine' that she heard things. This was an important step forward for her as it meant that she could recognise that the voices she heard came from her own imagination and therefore did not indicate that other people really thought badly of her. The dust explanation was also useful because she came to the conclusion that the medication that she had previously blamed for making her feel unwell could actually help to control the dust and therefore that it was worth taking for this reason. Interestingly, this girl was contacted in the community a year later, in connection with a CBT research project, and at this time it was found that she accepted that she had a mental illness and that this was what caused her to 'imagine' her voices. It was as if she had needed to modify her beliefs in stages, first by recognising that her voices did not come from a real person and only later being able to recognise that the cause of this false perception was internal (the illness) rather than external (the dust).

This latter case raises the question of whether one is colluding with a delusional explanation by helping the patient to use it to trigger appropriate coping strategies, and if so, whether this is acceptable practice from an ethical point of view. Although the primary aim of the therapist is always to reduce the patient's distress this may in some cases appear to conflict with the ethical standard of being honest and truthful with your patient, at least in the short term. In essence this is the 'paternalism' debate in a new guise. Should you take control of the situation and make the decisions in order to do 'what's best' for your patient or should you respect his right to take full charge over his own life even if that means a poorer outcome for him? In practice, it is a question of where you draw the line between two extreme positions and individual therapists will no doubt differ in where that line falls. You should be aware, however, that when making this decision you will almost certainly be basing it on your own beliefs and preferences and how you think you would feel in a similar situation. My own position in such cases is that whilst I would not suggest a partial insight explanation to the patient which I believed to be frankly untrue, I certainly would not seek to disprove any explanation that the patient had arrived at himself if it had beneficial effects for him, not least because this alternative explanation might be a stepping stone on the way to full insight.

In general, alternatives to the delusional belief that are untrue in fact are potentially vulnerable because there is always the risk that they will be shown to be wrong by subsequent events, so factually accurate alternatives are to be preferred for practical as well as ethical reasons. However, in seeking to achieve full insight with factually accurate alternative beliefs, you should be careful not to risk dislodging an inaccurate but functional partial insight until you are sure that the full insight explanation is the one that the patient will adopt in its place. In the case of inaccurate but functional explanations and beliefs, I recommend that you adopt a position of neutrality or ignorance about your patient's views if you do not want to change them, and in some cases even indifference to the explanation may be appropriate. For instance, in the 'dust' example given above, I took a stance along the lines 'I really don't know whether your voices are caused by the dust or not; I've never heard of that happening before but people can react differently to things, so who knows? I agree that the work we've done certainly indicates that the voices are not coming from the people whose voices they appear to be. But I don't suppose it really matters what's causing the voices, the only thing that is really important is to find out what you might be able to do to stop them when they are having a go at you'.

Caution: If you are working towards full insight but your patient seems to be more comfortable with a partial insight that attributes the symptoms to some other external cause rather than to something within himself, then you should be alert to the possibility that he may be unwilling to accept the explanation of mental illness because of the implications and stigma attached to that explanation. Therefore, whenever you feel this is a possibility, you should be sure to destigmatise the illness explanation (see later this chapter) before pressing on to achieve full insight.

A different type of partial insight occurs when patients deny having an illness but accept that other people genuinely believe that they are ill. In most cases the patient believes that other people are wrong in their beliefs about his illness, but nevertheless this level of insight allows him to accept that other people have good intent towards him when they treat him as if he were ill. However, we have observed in a number of patients, especially in those with long-standing illnesses, a rather peculiar partial insight where the patient seems to accept the truth of both his own belief that he is not ill and other people's belief that he is. It seems that these patients can move flexibly from one apparently conflicting belief to the other and act accordingly, without being affected by their incongruence. It is unusual for incompatible beliefs to be held together, without one being modified, but it may be that in these cases the evidence that the patient has to substantiate each of the beliefs is so convincing that neither can be rejected and so neither is able to take permanent precedence over the other. The maintenance of both beliefs may be enhanced by the fact that both can be functional for the patient in different contexts.

Be that as it may, this type of partial insight is useful in that it allows the patient to use coping strategies despite his denial of illness. For example, patients may continue to take their medication reliably, even when they are out of hospital and self-medicating, despite denying any need to do so or that they derive any benefit from it. When we first met with patients of this kind we thought that the most likely explanation for their treatment compliance was the power of the patient role in making them submissive to authority, but we no longer believe this to be so, certainly not in all cases. In some cases the patients seem genuinely to be able to behave according to two apparently directly opposing beliefs, without being aware of the incompatibility of those beliefs.

TOTAL VERSUS PARTIAL INSIGHT

The normal practice is to go for total insight as the goal of choice and only to resort to partial insight where total insight is not achievable, because full insight will be more stable than partial insight and less vulnerable to relapse. However, where the treatment goal of choice is a partial modification then it is likely that partial insight will also be the goal of choice. In these cases you should aim for the maximum level of insight that is possible without risking those parts of the delusional system that are to be kept intact. It might be possible to establish a partial insight that attributes the unwanted beliefs and hallucinations to 'illness' whilst leaving the beneficial beliefs and hallucinations unquestioned, but you would have to be very careful. As a general rule, the more similar the subject matter of the beliefs, the more likely it is that the insight gained about one belief will be transferred to the other; for example, it would probably be impossible to attribute some voices to 'illness' whilst leaving the patient with the comforting belief that other voices came from caring spirits. So where the delusional beliefs are similar in nature you should be particularly careful about the possible impact on one belief of the insight and modification work that you do on another. In some cases you may decide that it is not advisable to do any insight work at all about a delusion, even though it is an unpleasant one, because of the risk that the insight gained about the unpleasant delusion could transfer to and undermine other, beneficial beliefs.

WHEN INSIGHT IS NOT WELCOMED

Where the goal of choice is total insight, the insight promotion work seeks to make the patient aware that things and experiences he has previously attributed to the outside world or to outside agencies are actually produced internally, from within himself. You should not assume that this awareness will be a welcome one. If the experiences or beliefs are very unpleasant ones for the patient then it is easy to slip into the error of assuming that he will be delighted to discover that they are not true in fact. However, the positive effects of discovering that there is no basis in reality for his unpleasant experiences or fears may be comprehensively outweighed by the negative effects of realising that he is mentally ill. Most people have a poor understanding of mental illness in general and of schizophrenia in particular, so it should not be surprising if our patients also hold inaccurate or distorted beliefs, or fear the implications of such a diagnosis.

In order to ensure that the patient's new understanding about his symptoms and experiences will be helpful and comforting rather than distressing, the insight promotion work is done within a so-called 'normalising' framework. This seeks to modify the patient's beliefs about his illness and symptoms by a combination of education together with a reinterpretation or 'reframing' of the symptoms in terms of extremes of normal experiences. This latter way of conceptualising the symptoms, i.e. as being similar to normal experiences, as differing from normal experiences in degree rather than type, helps people to understand that having a diagnosis of schizophrenia does not mean that they are essentially different or set apart from 'normal' people, and furthermore that it is nothing to be ashamed or afraid of.

A guiding rule for insight promotion work is that you should always seek to ascertain your patient's understanding about mental illness and his attitude to having such a diagnosis before starting on the actual insight work. If his attitude is unfavourable then you must do the destigmatising work first. If perchance you are unable to successfully destigmatise the illness explanation then you should consider whether a partial insight might be more beneficial for the patient overall. Whenever there is any doubt about the patient's understanding or attitude it is safer to do some destigmatising work first. This may 'waste' time if it was not strictly necessary but it avoids the potentially serious risk of adverse reaction if the insight about having a mental illness or schizophrenia is abhorrent to your patient.

This lesson in better-safe-than-sorry was brought home to me with one of my earliest patients. This young man acknowledged that he had schizo-phrenia and attributed many of his strange experiences and beliefs to his illness and therefore I had not anticipated an adverse reaction to the work we were doing to modify another of his delusional beliefs. In between sessions he came to the sudden realisation that all his unpleasant experiences were probably illness related, which brought home to him the impact that the illness had had on his life. His immediate response to this overwhelming realisation was to take an overdose. Fortunately he was an inpatient and reported what he had done immediately, so he suffered no adverse effects from the overdose. Furthermore, I was able to see him without delay to help him to reassess the advantages and disadvantages of this new understanding, as a result of which he welcomed the greater insight he had developed and we were able to move rapidly on to tackle some of the other issues that had been worrying him. But although this case turned out well in the long run, it does demonstrate that you should never assume that your patient will view things as you do, or in the way you think you would view them if you were in his place.

THE INSIGHTS TO BE PROMOTED

Before moving on to look at some of the strategies one can use to help to promote insight within a normalising, destigmatising framework, it may be helpful to look at the sort of insights we are attempting to develop. A sample of these is given in Table 7.1. Note that we attribute delusional ideas and hallucinations to the patient's 'brain' and not to the patient himself. Since the patient does not willingly produce these phenomena, 'blaming' the brain rather than the patient for their occurrence is actually more accurate, as well as being preferable on the grounds that it avoids any overtones of personal criticism or devaluation of the patient for having them. Furthermore, this differentiation has proved useful in allowing patients to change their beliefs without undermining their self-esteem.

As with other aspects of CBT with schizophrenia, the following strate-gies that may be useful in helping to promote insight are not mutually exclusive and the order in which they can be included in a treatment programme is not fixed. Also, as with other aspects of CBT with schizo-phrenia, you would not expect to use all the possible strategies with any one patient. Usually you would expect to move from one strategy to another and back again, developing each strategy as the patient's overall level of insight increases. For example, it might be appropriate at an early stage just to note that from time to time many people hear voices that are not really there, and only later go on to draw the analogy between this and the patient's voices, and even later still explain how our brains might

Table 7.1 Useful insights for CBT with schizophrenia

Believing something to be true does not necessarily mean that it is true.

Because something seems obviously and evidently true does not necessarily mean that it is true.

Just because I intuitively 'feel' something to be true doesn't necessarily mean that it is true, however certain I may feel about it.

Believing something to be true that is not actually true is very common indeed, so it is not a weird or peculiar thing to do.

We all hold some beliefs that do not accurately reflect reality. We are not aware of their inaccuracy when we believe them. Holding inaccurate beliefs does not matter unless it causes us a problem.

It is OK/good to realise I was wrong about a particular belief and to change it accordingly.

We can imagine things that are impossible in the 'real' world.

Because I can imagine something happening does not mean that it will happen – nor does imagining it happening in any way increase the likelihood of it happening.

My brain is capable of misinterpreting things and giving me the wrong information.

Our brains are capable of producing very strange experiences; these experiences may be completely convincing at the time but completely wrong or even impossible in the 'real' world.

Anyone can get an 'odd' experience as a result of their brain not functioning accurately.

I am not 'weird' or peculiar if I hear voices – it's just an extreme of what happens to lots of people.

Hearing voices or having odd ideas only matters if they bother or upset me.

I can get an automatic thought about anything at all. Everyone's brain produces all sorts of automatic thoughts, including pleasant and unpleasant ones, sensible and silly ones. No-one can control what automatic thoughts come to their mind.

Therefore, I should not feel guilty or ashamed of the ideas that go through my mind or the beliefs that develop from them.

Similarly, I should not feel guilty or ashamed of what my voices say.

actually produce these hallucinatory experiences. The insight promotion work is closely tied in with and proceeds alongside the direct symptom modification work because increased insight can cause the patient to re-evaluate his delusional belief and work done to show that the delusional belief is not true can increase the patient's understanding about the nature of this belief.

STRATEGIES TO AID INSIGHT PROMOTION

These are summarised in Appendix 2.

DESTIGMATISING AND NORMALISING THE SYMPTOMS AND 'SCHIZOPHRENIA' LABEL

Whilst some patients readily accept that they are in hospital because they are ill and even that they have a mental illness called schizophrenia, others reject any such explanation as patently absurd and some react to the suggestion with horror. We have already noted that you should never assume that a patient believes and thinks about things in the same way that you do, however 'obvious' these things may be to you. Applying this maxim to the present context, do not assume that your patient realises that he has schizophrenia or even that he has a mental illness, even though he may have been in a psychiatric hospital for months or years, even though you may have heard other members of staff talking to him about his mental illness, calling it schizophrenia, and even though he acknowledges that other patients with him in the hospital or hostel do have schizophrenia. Certainly, the majority of patients in our unit, if asked why they are in hospital, will give some explanation that does not include mental illness. Some of the explanations I have heard recently include 'I needed a break', 'My flat needed cleaning and redecorating' and 'The hostel manager wanted to get rid of me'.

Some patients may have a distorted understanding of what is meant by schizophrenia so that even though they have some insight into their symptoms and recognise that they are ill, they deny that this illness could be schizophrenia. For example, one of our patients claimed that he could not have schizophrenia because he did not think that he was someone else, whilst another knew he did not have schizophrenia because he did not hear voices. Yet another of our patients had been terrified at being told she had schizophrenia because she thought this meant that she could go berserk and kill someone without warning. In these cases the promotion of insight would be aimed not only at increasing the patient's awareness of his symptoms but also at modifying his beliefs about what 'schizophrenia' means, with particular emphasis on what it means for him, both in terms of the present and the implications for the future.

Some patients may refuse to accept the diagnosis of schizophrenia because of the stigma attached to this label. This can be a difficult problem to deal with because it is unfortunately true that a large proportion of the general public do have an inaccurate and negative view of what the term means, often fearing that it implies irrational behaviour and unprovoked violence, so there is very real prejudice against people who are labelled 'schizophrenic'. In these circumstances the promotion of insight work aims to correct, develop and strengthen the patient's own awareness of what the term actually implies, with particular reference to his own case and symptoms, so that his beliefs about himself are strong enough to counter and reject the misinformed beliefs of others. The work also aims to strengthen his understanding that the negative beliefs and attitudes of others are based on their ignorance and are less accurate and knowledgeable than his own. Taking the role of expert helps to protect the patient's self-esteem against the prejudices of others and to protect his own beliefs from being undermined by the inaccurate beliefs of others.

Although it is not possible to change the beliefs of the general public at large, it can be very helpful to work with the immediate family and/or carers in order to modify any misconceptions they may have about the patient's diagnosis and what that implies for him and for them. Not only does this usually result in their adopting a more favourable attitude towards the patient but it also helps to reinforce and support the patient's own insights about his illness.

Modifying the patient's and carers' attitudes to the patient's schizophrenic illness is made harder by the fact that the end goal is for them to hold a different attitude and understanding about the illness from that held by the general public, so there is always the tendency for this latter to conflict with or even to reverse the beneficial changes being made. There is also the sad fact that even though the patient and his carers may come to regard his schizophrenia as nothing to be ashamed or afraid of, he may still be subject to the ignorance and prejudice of some people in the community and suffer accordingly.

Destigmatising the symptoms and reinterpreting them within a normalising framework is beneficial for most patients but it is essential preparatory work if the goal of the CBT is to enable the patient to discriminate and distinguish between thoughts, beliefs, voices, etc. that are due to 'illness' or 'brain dysfunction' and those that are not. It is essential to ensure that on gaining insight that these beliefs and experiences come from within himself he will understand that he is not weird, evil or morally reprehensible to have had them. The following strategies may be helpful in your attempts to normalise and destigmatise the patient's symptoms.

Sharing experiences of 'odd ideas'

This can be done in an individual therapy session or as a group discussion. The main purpose of this exercise is for you and/or your colleagues to share with your patient(s) any abnormal experiences you may have had. In this way you can demonstrate to him that having 'strange' experiences and ideas is actually quite normal, that he is not an 'odd ball' or member of some different species because he has them. You should, of course, acknowledge that your patient's experiences are probably more intense and disturbing than those of yourself or other staff, but the point is that they are different in intensity and effect rather than in kind. Sharing experiences with your patient not only demonstrates that it is normal to get strange ideas or feelings from time to time, but it also supports the key insight that feeling something to be so does not necessarily mean that it is so.

If you are doing this exercise with just your patient it may be helpful to share not only your own ideas and experiences but also those reported by other non-psychotic people. Given below are just some of the experiences reported by people on our CBT courses who have agreed that they may be shared with patients:

1. Entering a party and thinking that people had stopped their conversation in order to look at me.
2. A sudden panicky feeling that I was about to recover a 'lost memory' of having killed someone.
3. A conviction that the woman on the other side of the street was my mother who had died recently, so convincing that I followed her for several blocks.
4. Feeling convinced that other people in the room could read my mind.
5. Feeling sure that the plane would crash (which it didn't).
6. Swimming at sea and suddenly feeling that I could control the waves.
7. Fearing that my partner had left me on my own in the house because he had arranged for me to be murdered by a 'burglar'.

Since you are attempting to destigmatise mental illness, ideally you would share your odd experiences without hastening to explain them away; after all, the main purpose of the exercise is to demonstrate to your patient that he is *not* quintessentially different from you because he has these strange ideas and experiences. And bearing the purpose of the exercise in mind, the more psychotic-like the experiences that you share, the better! Whilst you should not feel under pressure to share a personal experience if you would feel uncomfortable in doing so, you should consider why you feel uncomfortable, as this may uncover some previously unrecognised belief or attitude in yourself.

Discussing the factors that increase vulnerability to 'odd ideas'

Discussing the circumstances in which delusions or odd ideas are more likely to occur in non-psychotic people helps to normalise the phenomenon by showing that, given the necessary conditions, anyone's brain can produce these psychotic-type experiences, i.e. it demonstrates that anyone can get 'odd' experiences as a result of their brain not functioning properly. This discussion can take place in a one-to-one therapy session or as part of a group exercise.

Patients may be able to make a connection between the factors that increase the brain's tendency to produce 'odd' ideas and the circumstances in their own lives when they experienced strange happenings and thoughts. For example, patients may recall being unable to sleep properly or being agitated or under stress before their hospital admission. As we have seen when considering partial insight, although attributing the symptoms to tiredness or stress is not entirely accurate, since it is probable that the tiredness and stress are caused by the same illness that also causes the delusions, nevertheless it can be a very helpful stepping stone on the way to insight as it does enable the patient to recognise his experiences as abnormal and also to explain them in terms of some physiological cause.

In non-psychotic people delusions are more likely to occur:

1. when under stress or anxious;
2. when depressed;
3. when ill with a high temperature;
4. when tired or sleep deprived;
5. when under the influence of street drugs or alcohol.

Education about automatic thoughts and the psychological processes involved in belief formation and maintenance

The purpose of this part of the insight work is for the patient to understand how the human brain works, so that he can understand why he gets the particular thoughts and experiences that he does and why his delusions are as they are. Further on into therapy, this work may be developed as the basis for his understanding of how CBT strategies can help to counter his delusions.

We have found that it is best to give this information as and when the opportunity occurs during therapy and in as much detail as the patient wants or shows interest in. We usually present the information as expert knowledge so that the patient does not feel ignorant for not knowing it already. Thus, we commonly use phrases like 'One of the things psychology has recently discovered . . .' and 'It's really interesting what scientists have found . . .'.

You may need to check from time to time to make sure that your patient has not picked up some distorted version of what you have tried to tell him; this is particularly likely to occur if you are not too sure of the facts yourself. Because it is important that you do not convey a distorted or confused understanding of this information to your patient it is important that you are clear in your own mind before you attempt to pass it on.

Automatic thoughts

You should share with your patient whatever information about automatic thoughts (see pp. 4–5) you think would be useful for him to have and you should present this in a way that he will be able to understand. Education about automatic thoughts usually includes the following.

1. Our brains are throwing up thoughts and ideas all the time, though we are not consciously aware of most of them.
2. It is functional for our brains to do this because it enables us to consider a whole range of possibilities, including possible interpretations of the present situation, possible responses and also the possible consequences of those responses.
3. Part of our brain selects out the most useful ideas and brings those into conscious awareness so that we can think about them more carefully.
4. Because our brains are throwing up these different ideas so rapidly it is not surprising that some of them are poorly formed, nonsensical or even completely wrong.
5. The unhelpful and poorly formed ideas normally drop out of our thought system straight away before we have become consciously aware of them, but occasionally our brain will latch on to one of them and give it more credence than it is worth.
6. Our automatic thoughts often reflect our worries and concerns, but they can be about anything at all, anything we have ever seen, heard or learnt about, anything we know about from any source at all.
7. We cannot control our automatic thoughts and therefore cannot be held responsible for them.

Responsibility for automatic thoughts – implications for guilt and shame

A very important aspect for CBT with delusions and hallucinations is the understanding that we cannot control the occurrence or content of our automatic thoughts and therefore cannot be held responsible or guilty for them. This follows directly from the more general argument that we cannot be guilty for what we cannot control. Most patients readily accept the truth of this general argument but if your patient has any doubts about it, then he must establish its truth first, before attempting to look at the issue of responsibility for automatic thoughts. Probably the easiest way of doing this is to use situations from everyday life, asking your patient each time if either he or a friend is guilty for what happened and if not, why not, bringing out the point that he is not guilty because he could not affect or influence the situation in any way. In the past we have discussed a number of events, including the execution of Anne Boleyn, the assassination of President Kennedy, the bomb planted at the 1996 Atlanta Olympics and the accident on the M1 last week, but others would do just as well.

Note: If your patient feels that he is able to influence events by some magical means, as may occur in some grandiose delusions, then you should go through these examples using a friend or some other person rather than the patient himself, or concentrate on historical events occurring before the patient was born.

Having established that we cannot be guilty for what we cannot control, it is easy to demonstrate the uncontrollability of our automatic thoughts by one or more of the following experiments.

1. Try to think of nothing at all for 30 seconds.
2. Try not to think of chocolate for 30 seconds.
3. Try to think only of chocolate for 30 seconds.
4. Try not to think about the pressure of the chair on your legs; think about anything else but not that.

Patients enjoy trying out these simple tests and they clearly demonstrate the point you are trying to make, namely that we cannot control our thoughts. It may be helpful to point out to your patient that we are no more able to control our automatic thoughts than we are to control the sensation of pain when our hand is pricked or to control the messages that our brain sends to our heart to keep it beating; our brain does all these things automatically and we just experience the results. Similarly, if, having achieved insight, your patient feels that he *ought* to be able to control his thoughts or hallucinatory experience, remind him that he cannot control the pain of an injection, even though he knows exactly what is causing it.

These exercises in attempting to control our automatic thoughts can also be useful in demonstrating that trying not to think of something may actually increase the likelihood of that thought coming to mind, because by trying to stop it we are inadvertently priming our brains to think about it. This may be helpful in explaining to your patient why his unwanted ideas or hallucinations may recur despite his recognition of what they are and his best efforts to keep them at bay. Also, unwanted ideas or hallucinations may recur because they produce a strong emotional response. This is true for all beliefs and experiences, not just psychotic ones. Anything that produces a strong emotional response in someone is likely to be potentially important for that person and so his brain is likely to bring it back to mind from time to time. Unfortunately, even when the patient has good insight about his delusional thoughts and hallucinations, the unpleasant or distressing material that they contain can still trigger a strong emotional response and so they are still likely to recur for this reason. Modifying the belief surrounding the material contained in the delusions and hallucinations is a major way of reducing the emotional response that they can cause and so this approach can also have a major effect on the frequency with which they recur (see Chapters 8 and 12).

One of the main reasons why people feel guilty and ashamed about their ideas and hallucinations is the widely held belief, probably stemming from misunderstood psychoanalytic theory, that our thoughts always reflect something about ourselves, so that even if they seem alien to us they nevertheless must be the product of our innermost longings and desires. It is often worth exploring this issue with your patient in case he has some underlying belief along these lines, in which case you should discuss the nature and role of automatic thoughts with him, noting that our automatic thoughts can reflect anything in our memories or knowledge systems and as such do not necessarily imply anything about ourselves or our wishes.

Another factor that may influence the patient's sense of responsibility for what is going through his mind is the fact that most of the thinking of which he is consciously aware will be under his conscious control and so he may assume that he must be responsible for *all* his thinking. If this is the case it may be helpful to clarify the difference between purposeful thinking and automatic thoughts, perhaps describing the automatic thoughts as the building blocks that are produced by the brain which can then be used or rejected by the more conscious and purposeful trains of thought. Whilst the latter is generally under the control of the person concerned, the former is not.

It may also be helpful if you draw a distinction between thoughts, the function of which is to suggest possibilities and offer options, and the actions that the person actually takes as a result of these thoughts. Thus, whilst we have control over our actions and as such are responsible for them, we do not have control over many of the thoughts that go through our minds.

Your patient may be reassured about the occurrence of his own antisocial or 'shameful' thoughts if you discuss with him the prevalence of such thoughts in the general population. For example, well over 50% of the population who have stood on a railway platform have had the thought of pushing a fellow traveller onto the rails, and it is quite common for car drivers to have the thought of driving on to a pavement and mowing down the pedestrians. You should point out that it is actually functional for people to have these antisocial thoughts because they warn them of what *could* happen. The fact that our platforms and pavements are demonstrably safe places to be indicates that thoughts are very different things from desires to act!

Whilst on the topic of antisocial thoughts in ordinary people, it may be helpful to consider with your patient what can happen when a mother has the thought of deliberately harming her own child, as an example of what can happen if there is a strong adverse reaction to an automatic thought. Most mothers will have had the thought at one time or another of deliberately harming their child, though very few ever carry it out in practice. Most women are able just to disregard the thought, without worrying about it, but a few feel so guilty and upset at having had such a thought that they keep thinking about it, leading to more emotional distress, leading to more thoughts about it and so on into a vicious cycle. This example may serve as a useful analogy to the recurrence of emotionally provocative hallucinations.

Intuitive thinking and jumping to conclusions

When talking with patients about their delusions we have found it very helpful to liken their delusional beliefs to intuitions, because intuitions are very normal occurrences that can and do happen to all of us. Intuitions are very similar to delusional ideas in that they can be based on very little or no objective evidence and yet they carry with them their own sense of conviction and certainty. Intuitions are also very similar to delusions in that although they can be accurate representations of reality, they are more often inaccurate and can be completely wrong, despite their feeling of correctness. Certainly some patients seem to find it more acceptable to think of their beliefs as inaccurate intuitions rather than as delusions, in which case this is the framework within which you should work. Your approach in this case would be along the lines 'Your brain seems to be particularly sensitive to intuitive thinking so it is likely to produce intuitions which will feel very true to you but that might not be true in fact. So it is important that you use the rational part of your brain to check out whether your intuitions are correct or not when you have them'.

Another 'normal' way of interpreting delusional ideas is to attribute them to the brain jumping to conclusions. As with intuitional thinking, jumping to conclusions is something that we all do and therefore is not stigmatising. The terms 'jumping to conclusions' and 'intuitions' have considerable overlap in meaning and usage, and in practice you will often find you use both terms with the same patient.

The two-route model of responding (see pp. 25–7) can be a useful aid in explaining to patients why they or their brains might have jumped to the wrong conclusion about something, or had a strong intuitional feeling, and why that could feel so convincing. If you are introducing this model to your patient you should first use it to explain how and why we jump to conclusions about things in everyday life, and how intuitions occur, and then extend it to include the patient's particular delusional ideas.

An example to illustrate the use of the two routes of responding in everyday life is someone walking along the road who hears a loud bang from just behind. The immediate response would be for the person to duck his head, put his arms up protectively and turn round – the rapid, immediate response of the subcortical route which has jumped to the conclusion that this may be a sign of danger. The slower but more thorough reasoning route would then evaluate the situation and respond according to the conclusions it reached and the options for action that were considered. For example, if the bang had come from an out-of-control car hitting a lamp-post then the likely considered response would be to take more effective protective action against the possible danger of being hit, perhaps by diving into a nearby garden, whereas if the bang had come from a workman knocking out the window of a house under repair then the likely considered response would be to straighten up and carry on walking. This illustrative example can also be used to show how the person's beliefs can influence the reactions and interplay of these two routes. For example, if the person believed that lonely streets are potentially dangerous at night then his immediate danger reaction would be stronger at night than if the same noise occurred in a busy street in the daytime.

An example you can use to illustrate the influence of our beliefs and fears on our intuitions and tendency to jump to conclusions is the not uncommon situation of someone about to board a plane who has the strong feeling that it will crash. In this case the intuitional feeling is reflecting an underlying fear about what *might* happen on the flight but it is experienced by the person concerned as an awareness of what *will* happen. The underlying fear has created such a bias in the person's interpretation of events, and probably even his interpretation of his own thoughts, that his brain has wrongly jumped to the conclusion that the feared crash will definitely happen. Once his brain has come to this conclusion it attaches to it a convincing sense of certainty which may be difficult to shift by logical reasoning.

It may be helpful for your patient if you can explain why this sense of certainty, once attached by the brain, can be so difficult to dislodge. It relates back to the function of the automatic route of thinking, which is to provide a better-safe-than-sorry response: because this response may have biological significance for the person concerned, e.g. protection from danger, it would not be in the person's best interests if this response could be easily overridden. Even the intuition about the plane crashing has some potential beneficial effects to the person concerned, because if the person cannot overcome this feeling of certain tragedy and refuses to board the plane then this guarantees that he does not take even the very small risk of being killed in an air accident. Of course, he may lose out on the gains of a successful business trip or the pleasures of a holiday, but he will not risk death.

We saw in Chapter 1 how, once beliefs are established, they influence the way in which we interpret events so that our interpretations are in keeping with our existing beliefs and also serve to reinforce them. It may be helpful to use one or more of the examples described in Chapter 1 to demonstrate to your patient that it is quite normal for the brain to distort evidence and to jump to conclusions in this way and so it is not abnormal for his brain to have distorted his interpretation of the facts so that they fitted in with his delusional beliefs.

Discussing the meaning of 'schizophrenia'

If the end goal of your therapy is for your patient to understand his psychotic experiences in terms of a mental illness called 'schizophrenia' then clearly it will be necessary for him to have an accurate understanding of what that term actually means for him, but even if you are only going for partial insight it may still be important to do some educational and destigmatisation work about the term because it is likely that your patient will be aware that other people are saying that he has schizophrenia, even though he disagrees with this statement.

The information about schizophrenia and the way that you give it will depend on your patient's level of insight into his psychotic experiences; as a general rule, the better his level of insight, the more direct you can be in your discussions. It is important, therefore, that you ask questions during the assessment interview(s) to ascertain your patient's knowledge of and attitude towards schizophrenia, as well as assessing his level of insight about his own psychotic experiences. Some of the questions you could ask would include:

1. 'Why are you in hospital? Why does your doctor say you are in hospital? Does your doctor say you have an illness? What is it called? Why does he say that? What is schizophrenia?'
2. 'Why are other people here in hospital? Do the staff say that the other people here have an illness? What is it? Why do the staff say that?'
3. 'Do you know anyone with schizophrenia? How do you know he's got schizophrenia? What are the symptoms of schizophrenia in his case? Is that a bad thing to have? Why? Would it be awful if you had schizophrenia? Why?'

If your patient has poor insight about his own experiences you should conduct the educational, normalising and destigmatising work over many sessions. As a general guide, introduce only one or two ideas at a time and only as much information as feels comfortable and natural as part of a topic of conversation that your patient may feel is of little interest or relevance for him. If he turns the conversation along a different tack then go with this rather than persisting with your own agenda; you can always

return to the topic on a future occasion. The art is
mation to your patient as part of a general conversa
ideas about a topic of general interest. In the early
important not to imply that you believe your patien
though later you can discuss what this would/does mean i

Even if your patient denies that he has a mental illness,
certainly have been told by other members of the mental hea
he has schizophrenia so it is very unlikely that you would nee
this possibility with him yourself. Your aim is to enable him to
connections between other people's symptoms, his own experiei   d
what his doctor/nurse is telling him, by making this conclusion less
alarming and more relevant to his own experiences.

The model of schizophrenia that we usually use with our patients is a
stress/vulnerability model which says that schizophrenia occurs as a result
of a combination of an innate vulnerability to develop the illness plus
stress factors that trigger the illness. According to this model, people
differ in their vulnerability to schizophrenia because of innate biological
differences in their brains, so that in some people relatively little stress
can be sufficient to set the illness off whereas in others it would take very
high levels of stress indeed to produce any of the symptoms, with most
people falling somewhere in between these two extremes. The stress can
be either mental (e.g. with major life events such as bereavement, divorce,
new home and job, etc.) or physical (e.g. illness, solitary confinement,
etc.). This model provides a framework within which the brain can be
seen to be responsible for producing the symptoms of the illness and also
prepares the way for the notion that medication may help by correcting
some biochemical imbalance in the brain.

It is important to point out in your discussions that schizophrenia is
not a single illness but is a general term used to cover a range of possible
symptoms, so that no two people with schizophrenia will be affected in
exactly the same way. Indeed, it is possible to have two people with the
diagnosis of schizophrenia who have completely different symptoms.

When talking about schizophrenia it will probably be helpful to concentrate on your patient's own particular symptoms, taking care to point out
that for him the diagnosis does not imply anything more than his experiences and symptoms. In particular, it does not mean that he will develop
any of the other possible symptoms given in the text books or that other
people with this diagnosis may have. You can also reassure him that
although his illness may recur in the future the typical course of the
illness is a fluctuating one rather than a progressive, worsening one.

If your patient held prejudiced beliefs about schizophrenia it may be
worth making explicit that schizophrenia is not a character or personality
defect or weakness, and furthermore that this diagnosis does not mean
that the person concerned is 'mad' or 'weird', and it does not imply that

may suddenly behave in a peculiar way or go berserk and make a violent attack on someone.

Many people seem to treat the diagnosis of schizophrenia as if it described some core, essential part of the person concerned, as if the illness invades and affects every part of that person. Indeed, there is an unfortunate tendency to blame everything on the illness once this has been diagnosed. It is as if once the patient has been diagnosed as having schizophrenia, he cannot lose his temper for any non-psychotic reason, or his neighbours can never really be unpleasant to him, etc. Because of this widely held attitude it is often worth pointing out to your patient that most of his brain and body still works perfectly normally, and it may be helpful to go through with him all the things that he still does just like everyone else, e.g. talking, walking, dressing, etc. It is also worth pointing out that it is only a relatively very small part of his overall brain functioning that sometimes works inappropriately.

EXPERIENCE IS NOT THE SAME AS FACT

We have already noted that a major problem with psychotic experiences is that they are perceived as being self-evidently true and that as human beings we are predisposed not to doubt what we believe to be 'fact'. Therefore, in order for people with schizophrenia to challenge their delusional beliefs, it is necessary for them first to recognise that this feeling of absolute certainty that something is true can be misleading or even downright wrong. One or more of the following approaches may help to demonstrate to your patient that perceiving something to be self-evidently true does not necessarily mean that it is true and that the brain can give misleading information about how things really are.

Misinterpretation of everyday events

We all can and do misinterpret events that happen in our everyday lives. Misinterpretation can occur at a perceptual level, resulting in misperception, or further along in the processing, at the level of event evaluation, as the following examples show.

1. I hear my neighbours next door having a furious row but later discover that it was a television programme they were watching.
2. I hear my friends criticising my new hairstyle but later discover they were discussing someone else.
3. I bend down to pick up a piece of mud on the carpet but discover that it is an ink stain.
4. I walk along and the moon in the sky seems to follow me wherever I go.

5. I pull my hand away sharply as an insect lands on it, but it was only a leaf.
6. I interpret the pain in my chest as a massive heart attack, but later realise it must have been indigestion.
7. I enjoy a slice of bread and butter, but later discover it was bread and a vegetable fat substitute (if the adverts are to be believed!).
8. My friend forgets to send me a birthday card, but I later discover that it was actually sitting in a postbox because of a strike.
9. I think that my daughter has done very well to get a grade 1 in her maths exam, until she tells me that the usual way of marking is reversed and 9 is the top grade.

These examples may seem very obvious and unremarkable but this makes them all the more useful in demonstrating that it is really quite common for us to be misled in our interpretation of events and situations, and that believing something to be so does not necessarily mean that it is so. To destigmatise these 'errors' and make them relevant to your patient, you should share any of your own experiences of this sort and also encourage your patient to recall any of his own from everyday life.

One of the important aims of the normalising and destigmatising work is to enable your patient to change his delusional belief without feeling that he must have been odd or stupid to have held this belief in the first place. As a general rule, the more important a belief is to us, the more firmly we hold on to it and the more vigorously we have defended it in the past, the harder it is for us to admit that we were wrong in that belief. Delusional beliefs are commonly of this type, so where your patient has invested time and energy in maintaining and defending his delusional belief it is particularly necessary to ensure that he can change this belief without feeling he has lost face or that his self-esteem is affected. Educational work around the formation and maintenance of beliefs generally – and/or sharing your speculations about how your patient's delusional belief might have arisen – will help him to understand that it was quite reasonable for him to have held the delusional belief, given the circumstances he was in and the experiences he was having.

Past beliefs no longer held

Sharing experiences of beliefs once held but now disavowed will demonstrate that believing something to be so does not guarantee that it is so. Furthermore, it is another way of demonstrating that it is perfectly normal to hold some 'incorrect' beliefs and therefore that we should not feel silly or stupid when we realise that they are incorrect or fear loss of face when we acknowledge our errors to other people. In our discussion groups, participants have reported the following firmly held beliefs which they now acknowledge to have been wrong.

1. Father Christmas visits each year with a sackful of toys.
2. The Tooth Fairy collects old teeth and leaves a silver coin in their place.
3. The Conservatives are the best party to govern Britain.
4. John Lennon was the most attractive man ever born.
5. The Turin shroud was Jesus' burial cloth.
6. My partner will never leave me and go off with someone else.
7. I will never feel happy again now that my partner has left me.

The discussion about inaccurate beliefs held in the past should also stress the normality of changing these beliefs once we know them to be wrong, and the advantages to us of doing so. This will support the notion that your patient is not unusual or stupid for holding a (delusional) belief which he later discovers to be inaccurate, and furthermore that it is perfectly normal and acceptable to change his belief.

   If your patient can recall any delusional beliefs that he held in the past that he now realises were delusions then these will provide very useful evidence not only that his brain is capable of holding inaccurate beliefs but also that the conviction he had in those beliefs at that time was totally misleading. Therefore, since feeling sure about something does not guarantee that it is correct, you can discuss why it would be beneficial for him to learn how to check out his ideas in the future, using his rational reasoning abilities, rather than relying on his feelings.

Misperception at a physiological level

This is particularly pertinent for insight into hallucinations and so is included in detail in Chapter 11, p. 181–3. This strand of the work can be useful for delusions because it demonstrates not only that the brain is capable of misperceiving things at the very basic level of the senses but also that it can continue to misperceive these things even though the person concerned knows rationally what the true state of affairs is.

Use of dream analogy

Everybody has experienced abnormal or bizarre events, perceptions, feelings, etc. in dreams so dreams are a very useful 'normal' equivalent of psychotic experiences. A major advantage of using this analogy is that dreams are totally convincing whilst they are happening and any inconsistencies, illogicalities, etc. are not appreciated until after waking. This may be used to strengthen the insight that because something seems obviously and evidently true at the time does not necessarily mean that it is true.

Since 'normal' brains can produce such strange yet convincing experiences of reality, and indeed do so regularly, this will support the suggestion that the patient's brain could also be responsible for producing some strange and convincing (but inaccurate) experiences whilst he is awake and therefore that this is a possible explanation for these experiences. Furthermore, it supports the notion that the patient's brain is not weird or essentially different from other people's brains in being able to produce these strange experiences.

Another major advantage of the dream analogy is its use to reinforce the conclusion from the educational work about automatic thoughts, namely that your patient should not feel guilty or ashamed because of the content of his delusions or hallucinations. Almost without exception, the patients we have worked with do not feel guilty about the content of their dreams, so assuming that your patient also holds this point of view you can use this to argue that, just as he is not responsible for the material produced by his brain during dreaming, neither is he responsible for what it produces during hallucinations or for the delusional ideas that come unbidden to his mind.

Of course, if your patient did believe that his dreams reflect his inner thoughts and desires then you could not use this particular line of argument with him unless and until you were able to modify his belief about dreams. The theory of dreams that we usually use is that dreaming is the brain's way of clearing out all the remnants of the previous day's unwanted thoughts and perceptions, so although they are likely to reflect the person's interests and concerns they do not necessarily do so in any accurate way.

Some patients use the dream analogy to make sense of their psychotic experiences, for example 'My brain sometimes acts as if it were dreaming, even though I am awake' or 'It was one of my waking dream experiences'. This way of interpreting the experiences may be particularly suitable for describing delusional memories but it can also be useful for hallucinatory experiences. The 'dream' interpretation emphasises the essential 'normality' of these experiences, because although it is not normal to experience such things when awake it is certainly normal to experience them whilst the brain is in sleep.

Imagination is not the same as reality

Some people with schizophrenia have particular difficulty discriminating between imagination and reality. One effect of this is that they imagine something happening and then assume that this means that it could happen, and indeed even that it is likely to happen. When this involves bad or unwanted events the thinking seems to jump from 'Wouldn't it be awful if...' to 'It's only a question of time until...'. If you note this to be a feature of your patient's thinking then it should be pointed out and discussed with him.

In order to demonstrate that imagining something happening does not increase the likelihood of it happening or even that it is possible for it to happen, you can ask your patient to imagine pleasant things that are unlikely to happen, for example winning the lottery or having champagne at supper, and to imagine events that would be clearly impossible in actual life, for example walking on the moon or jumping over a house or breathing under water, etc. It is usually easier for patients to see that imagination does not and cannot affect reality using pleasant images than with unpleasant images.

DISCUSSION OF HOW AND WHY THE DELUSIONS MIGHT HAVE OCCURRED

You cannot launch into a discussion with your patient about the possible origins of his particular delusional beliefs until he recognises that his ideas could possibly be inaccurate and, more commonly, you would not share your speculations with him until he had reached the stage of realising that his beliefs were very probably or definitely incorrect. The complexity/simplicity of the alternative explanations and perspective that you offer your patient should be adapted to his level of insight and his ability to understand.

When offering an alternative explanation for a delusional belief, you should always make very clear that this is only one possible explanation of how your patient's beliefs might have developed. Whether or not your speculation is correct in all particulars may not matter; the important thing is that it is reasonable and seems plausible to your patient. A principal aim of this part of the work is to anchor your patient in the objective, matter-of-fact world by showing him that it is perfectly possible to explain his beliefs and experiences in terms of the way he or his brain has misinterpreted ordinary events, that it is not necessary to resort to unlikely or esoteric explanations to account for them.

Giving your patient some alternative and acceptable explanation for why his delusional beliefs developed is important for long-term therapy because without such an explanation it is much more likely that, should the psychotic experiences recur in the future, the delusional belief will be accepted again. After all, if you feel that someone is trying to harm you it is not unreasonable to suppose that the most likely explanation for this feeling is that someone really is trying to harm you. So when the feeling came on you again that someone wanted to harm you, you would need to have a very solid alternative explanation for feeling this way to counter the more obvious and straightforward interpretation, namely that it was true.

Using the model for the formation and maintenance of delusional beliefs

We have found that the simplified working model described in Chapter 2 provides a useful and destigmatising framework that can be adapted to suggest possible alternative explanations for the individual patient's particular delusional beliefs. If your patient recognises that he has a mental illness, i.e. that his experiences are somehow related to part of his brain not functioning properly, then this model helps to explain why his brain could have produced the sort of experiences and ideas that he has had.

The inclusion of biosocial systems into the model for delusions is still speculative but it has two definite advantages for the patient. First, it provides him with a biological explanation of why he might feel something to be so even though it is not actually so, for example why he might feel paranoid even though no threat to him actually exists. Second, it provides an explanation for his feelings and delusional beliefs in terms of an overactive or oversensitive response from an otherwise normal brain function; for example, it could explain the feelings of paranoia in terms of an oversensitive activation of the body's alert-to-danger system. Explanations in terms of inappropriate triggering of normal psychological systems are likely to be less alarming and less stigmatising for the patient than the notion of 'abnormal' functions or madness.

It is not necessary to introduce the notion of biosocial systems into your explanation unless your patient has reached the stage of wanting to know exactly how his brain could be misfunctioning, and indeed it is not even necessary to use the notion of mental illness when you use this model. If your patient is still cautious about accepting that he has schizophrenia then you can still use the model to explain his delusional experiences but starting from the mood/feeling stage. For example, your explanation might run along the lines of 'For some reason a mood or feeling that would normally be produced in response to external events just occurred, without anything in the outside world actually having happened to cause it . . .' – and then carry on to explain what could happen after that feeling had occurred. The advantage of linking the mood/feeling that is driving the delusional belief to some sort of brain malfunction, even if the nature of this malfunction is not explored, is that this paves the way for and supports the idea that medication could help to correct and prevent whatever it is that is causing the delusional ideas.

Example from clinical practice

One of my patients asked me why she would *think* that people were insulting her when they used the 'ě' vowel sound if they were not really doing so. This belief caused her a lot of distress in everyday life. It was also having an adverse effect on other aspects of our therapy because I would use the 'ė' sound many times during our sessions and despite my efforts to consciously control them I would inevitably stress a number of these (I discovered that it is particularly easy to emphasise the 'ė' when replying 'Yes' to a question). So we were constantly having to stop what we were doing to challenge this interpretation of my speech each time it occurred. We had used several different ways to challenge the validity of her underlying belief and these were sufficiently successful in instilling doubt in her mind to enable her to ask me what other explanation there could be for her feelings of being insulted other than the obvious one that people were really insulting her. She was already aware that she had schizophrenia and that this made her feel paranoid, though like many patients with good insight into their illness she denied that this particular belief could be part of that illness. But the fact that she knew that she had a paranoid illness meant that this could be incorporated into our suggested model of how this particular belief could have arisen, a model that accounted for her belief in terms of factors that did not include that people were really trying to insult her.

The patient found diagrams helpful, so the diagram given in Figure 7.1 was constructed. The explanation that accompanied the presentation of this model ran along the following lines.

'You have an illness that makes you feel threatened and persecuted. That's what you take your medication for but, as you know, unfortunately this doesn't completely control your illness so there will be times when you feel threatened and persecuted, not because anything threatening or dangerous has actually happened, but just because that's the way your illness makes you feel. Once the danger-warning system in your brain has been alerted then it looks to see what might have caused it to be alerted, and since danger normally does come from outside of us, it is perfectly reasonable for the brain to look to the outside world for the source of that danger. It doesn't do this consciously, of course, it's at a much more basic, instinctive level than that. So at this basic, automatic, instinctual level your brain is trying to work out who or what is posing the threat, and how. Supposing all this happened at some time when you were sitting in a room talking to somebody. Now our brains are biased towards interpreting people or animals as more likely sources of threat than things like tables and chairs, because in real life people are indeed more potentially dangerous than inanimate objects, so in this case if there was one other person in the room then it would be perfectly reasonable for your brain to fix on

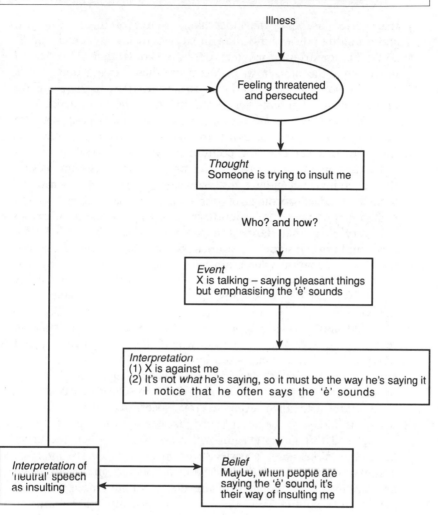

NOTE

The more this happens, the more likely you are to jump to the conclusion that you feel threatened because people are using the 'è' sound. In this way the belief is built up.

Now that you have the belief that people using the 'è' sound means that they are putting you down this will **confirm** your belief that emphasising these sounds is a way people use to insult you; just hearing someone emphasising those sounds may be enough to make you feel threatened.

Fig. 7.1 Possible explanation of why you gradually developed the belief that using the 'è' sound meant that people were trying to insult you.

that person as being the most likely source of threat. But you still wouldn't know how this threat was being signalled and it could be important for your brain to know that in order to judge what the danger was. Again, in these circumstances it is not unreasonable for your brain to suspect that if there are no physical signs of threat then the threat must lie in what is being said. Suppose, when all this happens, that the person you are talking to is saying pleasant things. If he is saying pleasant things then it can't be the content of what he is saying that is indicating threat. But perhaps you notice that he is emphasising the 'è' sounds when he talks. We have already seen, when we looked at tape recordings of our own conversations, how often people emphasise the 'è' sound when talking to one another, so it is very likely that the person you were talking to at that time was emphasising some 'è' sounds. So maybe, in this situation, the best explanation your brain can come up with as to why you have been 'threatened' is that it must be in the way the other person stresses the 'è' sounds. Once your brain has jumped to this conclusion, it is not unreasonable for you to develop the idea that maybe when people are saying the 'è' sound it is a sign that they are trying to put you down. If this feeling occurs again when you are in a social situation then you have an immediate explanation for it, i.e. the idea that when people stress the 'è' sound it's a sign that they are insulting you. Once this belief has been established then even neutral speech containing the 'è' sound is likely to be interpreted as being insulting or threatening, and this interpretation will serve to strengthen the belief about the 'è' sound. It's perfectly normal for people to interpret a situation in terms of their existing beliefs, so once your brain had assumed that people stressing the 'è' sound was a sign that they were insulting you, then it was perfectly understandable why you interpreted subsequent situations according to this belief. But unfortunately, these misinterpretations will have reinforced the incorrect belief, and so it got stronger rather than weaker.'

We were also able to use this diagram to explain how CBT might be able to help to combat these unpleasant feelings and the role that medication had in controlling them. Medication was shown to act on the 'illness' part of the model and this explained why it could help stop the feelings of persecution that were caused by the illness, whilst CBT was shown to act on the maintaining belief/interpretation cycle and this explained why it could help stop the feelings of persecution that were caused by the inaccurate/delusional belief.

This model was also used to explain to the patient why we thought it would not be a good idea for her to attempt to control her symptoms by CBT alone. Although CBT could combat the unpleasant feelings produced by the delusional beliefs and misinterpretations, it could not get rid of those that were caused directly by the biological activity of the illness. Only some biological intervention, such as medication, could do that.

Using the two-route model

The two-route model described in Chapter 2 is particularly relevant and useful for patients who acknowledge that their beliefs are based on a sense of inner certainty rather than on any hard objective evidence (e.g. 'I just know that it's true') and for patients whose beliefs are based on delusional feelings of significance (e.g. 'I was suddenly aware that his green tie had a special significance for me'). The two-route model does not involve the notion of mental illness, and even the implication that the brain is not functioning entirely normally is not strong, so it can be very useful for people with poor insight or who are reluctant to accept a diagnosis of mental illness. The model provides a way of explaining to people why their self-evidently true beliefs could be mistaken, despite their feeling of certainty, using the very normal and non-stigmatising notion of intuitions and the brain's tendency to jump to conclusions.

The two-route model also provides a very simple way of explaining to your patient what CBT is attempting to do, namely to use his reasoning, rational route of thinking to counter the more automatic, intuitional route. In order to reinforce the notion that your patient should follow his rational thinking rather than his intuitional thinking when the two come to different conclusions, it may be helpful to talk about the rational route as the higher or superior route and the intuitional route as a lower, more basic or animal way of responding.

When explaining the two-route model to your patient you should first describe how the two routes work in everyday life. In doing so you should explain why, for the most part, it is a good thing that we have this rapid all-or-nothing way of responding, because this allows us to take action very quickly in response to a situation where a rapid response may be more important than an entirely correct one. You should also explain why it is functional for the brain to respond in a better-safe-than-sorry way, namely because it is better to take cover when there is no danger than to risk not taking cover if danger actually exists. These explanations may help your patient later to understand why he jumps to the sorts of conclusions and develops the sorts of delusional beliefs that he does.

Example from clinical practice

The following gives you an example of how you might use the two-route model illustrated on p. 26 to give your patient an alternative explanation for his beliefs, and how the model can provide a rationale for using cognitive techniques to challenge some of the conclusions that he reaches.

'We've had a look at the way our brain uses two ways of thinking about situations in everyday life and how it usually uses both ways before coming to a final conclusion. There's the lower, more instinctive route that provides a very rapid conclusion, which can be helpful but which may not be accurate, and then there's the higher, reasoning route that takes longer to come to a conclusion but that is more accurate because of all the extra, high-quality thinking that has taken place. Although the lower route can be inaccurate, remember we noted how it gives the person the feeling that the conclusion it has come to is correct, and indeed it needs to do this in order to make sure that the person will react rapidly. It may be important that the person doesn't dither in his response so the brain has to make sure that he feels certain that it is the correct thing to do. The use of this route and the feelings of certainty that it brings happen to all of us, though in some people the feeling of certainty seems to be stronger than in others. Also, this automatic route seems to be more active in some people than in others; some people seem to have more of these intuitional ideas than other people. From what we've talked about before, it looks as though you might be one of those people who gets lots of intuitional ideas – what do you think? This might account for why you felt so certain that the drinking water was poisoned even though, when you looked for it, you could find no evidence to suggest that this was so. If your lower route was working overtime, this might also account for why you suddenly felt that the green tie worn by your doctor had special significance for you, even though your higher, rational thinking could not pinpoint what that significance was or find any evidence of a hidden meaning for it. But it's good that you know that your brain is particularly sensitive to intuitional ideas because that means that you can now be on the alert to detect them and to check them with your reasoning route. I know when we looked at this before, you concluded that if your reasoning route couldn't find any evidence or reasons to support a conclusion you had come to then you would know that this must have been the result of your intuitional route working overtime. And as your reasoning abilities are superior to the more basic, automatic responses of the brain, you know to rely on the former. Remember, don't be put off by the feelings of certainty that you get about a conclusion, because you know that where this is not supported by evidence, the feeling of certainty must have been produced by this lower route of responding and as such can be misleading. It will not be easy to counter such strong feelings of certainty as you get, but we'll be trying to find as many ways as we can to strengthen your rational route.'

Note on the use of models and flow diagrams

Whilst it is good practice to share with your patient as much of your own understanding about his symptoms and experiences as you can, do not assume that flow diagrams, even apparently straightforward ones, will necessarily make sense to him. Most of us working in the mental health field take diagrams for granted because we have learnt to use their symbolism during our training, but people without this familiarity may feel uncomfortable with them. If your patient is more confused than helped by a diagram then you should try to explain the same thing in words instead. However, even if you do not intend to share your diagram with your patient you may find it useful to formulate your own ideas in this way because it may help to clarify your thinking about the relevant factors involved and, equally important, it may help to expose gaps in that thinking.

8

CBT with the non-psychotic beliefs influencing the delusions

INTRODUCTION

Delusional beliefs, like any other new beliefs, are influenced in their development by the patient's existing network of beliefs (see pp. 7–9). In some cases the relevant belief(s) influencing the delusional belief will also be delusional, for example the patient who knew he was famous as a pop star because he had heard the presenter talking about him on the TV pop show the night before. Where one delusional belief backs up another in this way they are both targeted for modification, using the strategies described in Chapter 9. However, in many cases the relevant belief(s) influencing the delusional belief is not itself delusional, but nevertheless its modification may be an effective way of helping to control the delusional belief. Indeed, modification of a closely associated non-delusional belief may be the only way of ensuring a stable and permanent change to the delusional belief itself. If a non-psychotic belief is targeted for modification because it is supporting or strengthening a delusional belief, then it is usual to work on the modification of this belief at the same time as working on the delusional belief itself. The same approach and strategies are used to modify a non-delusional belief as are used to modify a delusional one (see Chapter 9).

The only time you would not consider modification of a non-delusional belief that was supporting a delusional belief would be if the non-delusional belief was otherwise appropriate and functional for the patient. For example, one of our patients believed that the police were pursuing him and waiting to pounce on him to put him in prison for a child sex offence that he had committed many years before. Although modifying his belief that the offence he had committed was punishable by prison would have helped reduce his delusional fear of being followed by the police, this modification was not done for two reasons. First, the belief was accurate and therefore an appropriate one to hold and second, the belief was one of the factors helping to prevent his re-offending.

In most cases the patient readily expresses the underlying beliefs that are influencing his delusional belief, but in some cases these underlying beliefs are not so obvious and so you should always be alert for clues as to their presence and content. One of the most useful clues is if there is a persistent theme running through the patient's different delusions. For example, in the case of the young man who believed he was mocked by strangers in the street it was noticed that these strangers were always young and female: it turned out that he believed he was sexually unattractive to the opposite sex, a belief that was providing strong support for his delusional belief. If they are not apparent, you may be able to elicit the associated beliefs by asking your patient about his delusion. For example, if the delusional belief involves other people you might ask him how he knows that these particular people are involved, why they would be involved rather than other people and why they should want to act in that way. This simple approach was useful for one of our patients who had a record of occasional violence towards other residents for which there was no apparent reason. During therapy he complained that one of his fellow residents was deliberately trying to provoke him and that if he carried on then he would have to hit him. When asked why this particular patient should want to do this, he explained that it was because this resident was an Irish Catholic. When asked about Irish Catholics, a number of dysfunctional beliefs were revealed, including that they were jealous of Ulster Protestants (the group to which the patient belonged) and that they wanted to take the material wealth that the Protestants were entitled to. On going back over his history, it was found that most of the people who had been hit by this patient were of Irish descent. It was not expected that modifying this patient's beliefs about people with Irish accents would weaken his feelings of paranoia *per se*, but it would be effective in removing a major reason why some particular people might be perceived as deliberately trying to provoke him.

The non-psychotic beliefs that are most likely to influence delusional beliefs include social prejudices (e.g. about race, gender, sexual preference, position in society and secret/security organisations), religious beliefs, moral beliefs and, in recent years, beliefs acquired from the world of science fiction and fantasy.

RELIGIOUS BELIEFS

Religious beliefs tend to be strongly held and exert a powerful influence over other beliefs, which have to be adapted to fit in with the religious beliefs. Religious beliefs are unusual in that there is general acceptance that they cannot be proved in the way that other beliefs about the world can be proved (hence the importance of faith) and therefore that they cannot be challenged as other beliefs can be challenged. No doubt this is one important reason why so many different religions exist in the world and why we are so far from reaching any kind of consensus on such fundamentally important issues.

If your patient holds what appears to be a delusional belief about a religious matter, it is essential that you ask him about his current religious beliefs and ascertain what the predominant religious beliefs were in his upbringing. This information is essential for you to evaluate whether the belief expressed is delusional or not, taking your definition of a delusion in this context to be any idea differing significantly from what is acceptable within that person's cultural and social group. For example, the belief that your dead parents are watching your every move would be delusional for someone brought up in a Western, Christian culture but not for somebody brought up in a culture that accepts the omnipresence of the spirits of the dead. Belief modification would be appropriate in the former case but not in the latter. Information about the patient's religious background may also be necessary to understand how the belief might have developed in the way that it has and what other underlying beliefs might be driving or influencing it.

Example from clinical practice

An elderly patient feared he was condemned to burn in the eternal fires of hell because he had masturbated when younger – understandably he was extremely distressed at this prospect. There were two significant beliefs involved in this delusion: first, that it was such a terrible sin to masturbate that it carried the worst possible sentence and second, that hellfire existed to give eternal torment after death. Theoretically, it should have been possible to remove the patient's fears and distress by eliminating either of these beliefs, because if it was not a sin to masturbate then he would not be condemned to hell even if hell existed, or if hell did not exist, then he could not be punished in this way however sinful the act of masturbation.

As the belief about masturbation being sinful is so unusual in our modern society, it was likely to be relatively easy to shift whereas his belief about hellfire, whilst much less common now than it used to be, has some strong advocates within our religious culture and as such was likely to be harder to change. The problem with tackling the belief about masturbation whilst leaving the belief about hellfire intact was our concern that, under the influence of the fear of hellfire, the patient might distort the evidence and find another reason why he could be condemned to this torment after death. In these circumstances it was undoubtedly safer to modify both beliefs, the 'delusional' belief about masturbation and the 'non-delusional' belief about hellfire.

Ethical considerations around the modification of religious beliefs

The example just considered raises an interesting and important question that particularly affects delusions involving religious and moral beliefs. In this particular case, should the patient's belief about the existence of hellfire be modified because it is dysfunctional for him in the distress it causes, or does it reflect some fundamental religious truth that should not be ignored or denied however unpleasant and whatever the personal cost? Because we tend not to question our own beliefs ('Of course they're true, I wouldn't believe them if they weren't!') there is a very real risk that the therapist may impose his own religious and moral beliefs on the patient through unwittingly selecting goals for therapy that are consistent with his own rather than the patient's core beliefs. Apart from being constantly on the alert for the possibility of this happening, there are two guidelines that you may find useful.

First, where there are alternative opinions or beliefs on a particular religious matter that are acceptable within the patient's religion and cultural background, you can consider modifying the patient's dysfunctional belief to one of the alternatives if that would be beneficial for him. For example, in the case mentioned above, since there were different views within the patient's religion (i.e. Christian) about whether or not hellfire exists, and since a belief in hellfire was so devastating for the patient, we set the goal for modification of his belief about hellfire to be that it does not exist. The patient was not attached to any church or denomination so this goal did not contradict any belief important to the socio-religious group to which he belonged.

The second guideline is to set the goals of modification in line with the central, generally accepted practice of the patient's religion. As a general rule, the beliefs of the more popular forms of the major religions tend to be more moderate and less judgemental than the minority, extreme sects. Furthermore, their wide acceptance amongst the people the patient mixes with means that they have a better chance of being reinforced by his day-to-day social contacts.

It is always much harder to work with a set of religious beliefs that are other than your own. Even if you know the main tenets of that religion you are unlikely to appreciate the relative importance of different aspects of the religion or the different shades of opinion that exist within it and, perhaps equally importantly, you are unlikely to understand the different ways in which people of different religions can think about these issues. For these reasons, wherever possible you should have access to ministers or elders of the main religious faiths who can advise you on the beliefs of their particular religion, and on what are considered to be acceptable shades of those beliefs within that religious group.

It may be helpful to call in a minister to talk directly with your patient if he is concerned about religious issues. We have been fortunate in our unit to have had access to ministers who are down to earth, non-dogmatic and non-judgemental, which are just the characteristics you want for this work, but ministers do vary greatly in their approach to religion so you do need to be careful that the minister's intervention will be helpful for your patient and not reinforce his delusions. For example, if your patient heard condemning voices that he believed came from the devil, it might not be helpful to call in the minister who regularly gave his parishioners messages from the spirit world during his services, or if your patient believed he was possessed by a ghost, it might not be helpful to call in the minister who believed in spirit possession.

Some fringe religious sects can hold extreme and rigid beliefs that can compound the suffering of people with schizophrenia and in these cases we tend to set the goals of belief modification away from those of the sect and nearer to those of a less extreme form of the core religion. For example, one of our patients would become very distressed after being visited by members of a Christian sect who would pray with her and then tell her that if she was still ill it was because she was not praying hard enough. I do not doubt for one moment that this advice was lovingly given, that her visitors genuinely believed this to be the case and therefore that this advice was in her own best interests, but nevertheless it left our patient not only suffering from some very distressing symptoms of her schizophrenia but also with a feeling of guilt that it was her fault that she felt this way because she did not love God enough. In this case, we did feel it was appropriate to challenge these particular religious beliefs and to modify them towards the more generally held views within the Christian religion about illness and prayer, and the hospital chaplain was extremely helpful in taking the patient through these issues with an authority on religious matters that we did not have.

We have also had a couple of cases where the patients' delusions about being condemned to eternal suffering have been exacerbated by feelings of guilt about leaving a religious sect. If the patient is religiously minded then a non-religious alternative belief will probably not be powerful enough to counter the fears associated with the sect's belief and therefore an alternative religious belief is a better aim. In such cases we would go for a belief that was in keeping with a mainstream version of the patient's current religion. For example, one of the factors supporting a patient's belief that she was guilty of a great sin was that she had left a religious movement some years earlier and therefore was no longer able to pray for the world's salvation as she had been taught she ought to do. She had been brought up in the general Christian religion of a non-churchgoing family but religion and religious issues were of a genuine concern and importance for her and so it would have been inappropriate, as well as probably ineffective, to attempt to remove her belief about the absolute authority of the religious sect without replacing it with some other belief that would make sense of her religious concerns. In this case, too, we called in the hospital chaplain who was able to use his beliefs about prayer and salvation to counter and modify the patient's dysfunctional beliefs.

MORAL BELIEFS AND VALUES

Similar considerations to those around religious beliefs apply to moral beliefs, though in practice these latter present less of a problem for the therapist because there is much more general agreement within our multi-ethnic society about core moral values than there is about religious truths. Probably for that reason, it is also more permissible within our society to question someone's moral beliefs and standards than it is to question their religious ones. One area of morality where there are still very different views, however, which can be passionately held, is that of sexuality and sexual behaviour. There are other contentious areas, of course, such as abortion, animal experimentation and conservation, but these tend not to occur in delusional beliefs.

In general, you would adopt a similar approach to goal setting and belief modification with morality as you would with religious beliefs, namely looking to find what belief would be most functional for the patient to hold within the range of beliefs acceptable to his cultural/social group. Note that it is not your role to change your patient's belief about a moral or social issue so that it conforms with the politically correct view. Because your patient is living within society, the current 'politically correct' belief may well be the most functional one for your patient to hold, but if it is not, then your role is to modify his belief to whatever is more functional for him even if this conflicts with your own views.

BELIEFS BASED ON TECHNOLOGY AND SCIENCE

Scientific and technological developments have progressed so quickly in the past few decades that it is not surprising that we understand little about some of the things that we use in our everyday lives. Where there is poor understanding of how things actually work it is easy for wrong explanations and extrapolations to be accepted as true. For example, most people have only a general understanding of what communication satellites do and an even vaguer understanding of how they do it, so it is not surprising that one of our patients could develop the delusional belief that the so-called spy satellites could see him in his room and send messages about what he was doing. Similarly, given the advances in organ transplant surgery, it is understandable that one of our patients could develop the delusional belief that all her digestive organs had been removed during an operation some years previously.

Modification of delusions that are based on inaccurate beliefs about the real world can be strengthened by exploring with the patient how the subject matter of the delusion really works, looking at what it can and, more importantly, what it cannot do in real life, and why it is limited in this way. For example, in the first of the above cases, we looked at how the space satellites work and what sort of thing they can detect, and in the second, we looked at how transplant surgery works and what the digestive system does. The valid, scientific explanation for how something works is the best alternative for a delusional explanation because, being true, it will be consistent with and therefore supported by other evidence from the real world. In such cases, you should provide your patient with as much detailed information as he needs or wants in order to form his new belief, which may well mean that you will have to hunt out the appropriate information from books or from people working in these areas. Ideally, you would encourage your patient to seek out this information for himself, on the grounds that what he discovers for himself is likely to be more persuasive than what you tell him, but in practice you will often have to do at least the preliminary research work to find the sources of the information he wants. It is likely that for your clinical work you will need to know how the TV system and surveillance cameras work, as these particular areas often feature in people's delusions.

BELIEFS BASED ON SCIENCE FICTION

It is known that delusional beliefs tend to follow the fashion of the times, reflecting the cultural experiences and values that are operating in society. For example, the demystification of royalty is probably responsible for the reduction in delusions of grandeur featuring royal connections whilst the rise and fall of such organisations as the KGB and IRA can be seen reflected in the content of patients' paranoid delusions. In recent years the popularity of science fiction and fantasy novels, and the ready availability of these ideas through films and television, have made a significant impact on the delusional beliefs developed by patients.

Ideas depicted in science fiction and fantasy range from the scientifically possible (e.g. life on another planet) to the frankly absurd (e.g. becoming very small and travelling round someone else's bloodstream). The problem with this area of fiction is that it does not discriminate for the reader or watcher what is feasible and what is not. Without this guidance, and without a basic scientific understanding of the world on which to judge the ideas portrayed, it is easy to see how people could conclude that even the most fantastic things are at least possible.

People may confuse fact with fiction if they are unable to recall where they learnt of a particular idea, so that ideas depicted in a science fiction story may be inappropriately recalled as something learnt as scientific fact. Delusional ideas that clearly break the laws of science (e.g. shrinking to a fraction of one's real size or being beamed to another planet) can be challenged using the laws of science to refute them. However, one of the most useful levers against a delusional belief based on a sci-fi story is knowing where it comes from, because this gives you the best chance of targeting your challenge to knock out the positive evidence on which the belief was based. So if you are not up on the popular sci-fi works and programmes it is helpful to have access to someone who is, who may be able to suggest where the ideas could have come from. One of our therapists was a sci-fi fan and she was able to help us identify the possible source of a number of different delusions, generating hypotheses that could then be explored with the patients. It was surprising how often she could come up with a possible basis for the strangest ideas!

We have noticed that some patients seem to make a poor distinction between what they see on films or TV and real life, so that if they have seen something on TV then they take this as good evidence that it could happen in real life. A few patients hold the even more extreme belief that if they have seen something on television or at the cinema then it *must* have happened that way in real life, on the not unreasonable grounds that otherwise the cameras would not have been able to record it happening as it did. Should this occur, the best way to counter such a belief is to describe what happens on a film set or TV studio and how scenes of things impossible in real life can be created. It may be helpful to describe how a film set might look, helping your patient to imagine the actors taking up only a small part of the studio and being surrounded by cameramen, directors, producers, make-up artists, etc. whom you cannot see on the film itself but who were there when the action portrayed was actually happening; for example, you know there must have been at least two cameramen present to take the film from the different perspectives.

Most patients are familiar with cartoon films and how they are constructed so this is a good example of how the end result of a film can be misleading. For example, it may look as if the mouse changes shape as it squeezes through the keyhole and pops out the other side, but of course, it is only really a set of different but unchanging flat, 2D pictures. Similarly, you can describe how other trick photography can make impossible things seem to happen. If you know the film or TV programme that your patient is using to support his delusional belief then describing how the effects might have been obtained and what the film set might have looked like whilst it was being shot may help your patient to re-evaluate the 'evidence' and hence the delusional belief it sustains.

Example from clinical practice

A patient feared that he would turn into a wild animal. After some discussion, it was agreed that his major piece of evidence that this was possible was a frightening and convincing film in which this had happened. We started by looking for any evidence of any other creatures turning from one thing into another and back again and used evidence and logical reasoning to argue that this could not possibly happen. We noted that the only dramatic transformations that seem to occur in nature were in the insect kingdom (e.g. a caterpillar changing into a butterfly) though even in these cases the insect was unable to return to its original form. We discussed how living bodies are basically made up of very complicated chemicals and that the molecules of chemicals cannot change unless something makes them change, which is usually the addition of other chemicals. We discussed how the molecular structures of hair and flesh are very different, so a cell of hair cannot change into a cell of flesh and vice versa. We discussed how the insect transformations occurred, with new cells developing and gradually replacing the old cells, rather than the old cells changing into the new ones. We noted that even the most rapid insect transformations would take a day to occur and therefore that this would imply that for any similar significant change of shape to take place in a human, who is at least 50 000 times heavier than an insect, this would take over 136 years to achieve – certainly a lot longer than the few seconds it had taken on the film! We also noted that the beast he feared changing into was much heavier than a human so a lot of extra biological material would have to appear out of nowhere, and it was explained why this could not happen according to one of Newton's laws of physics (the conservation of energy/matter). Similarly, a lot of biological material would just have to disappear again when the beast changed back to a human, and again it was explained why this was equally impossible according to the laws of physics.

Having prepared the ground by working directly on the patient's delusional belief, we then moved to discredit the major piece of evidence he had to support this belief, namely his assumption that because he had seen the transformation from man to beast in a film on TV it must have happened like that. For this aspect of the treatment the appropriate goal was to modify his belief that his eyes could not deceive him and in particular, his assumption that what he saw on TV had necessarily happened at some time in the past because otherwise it could not have been filmed. This latter was done by explaining how the scene had probably been made, with a series of small changes to the man's make-up being made, with more bits of fur being added each time, and separate photos shot at each stage of the procedure. We noted that this would probably have taken hours to do in real life, with most of the time being taken up by the make-up girls adding bits of rubber and fur to the actor's face and changing his costume for each shot, so that although it had actually taken hours to make it was presented as just a few seconds for the film, with none of the busy activity that had taken place in the studio being shown. The patient knew about cartoon films so the apparent transformation that had taken place was likened to the laborious process of building up a cartoon film.

CONCEALED BELIEFS

Delusional ideas may be associated with underlying beliefs that are not immediately apparent and only emerge during therapy. You should consider the possibility of an undetected underlying belief:

1. if there are aspects of the delusional belief that you cannot account for in your speculations about why the delusion might have developed in the way that it has;
2. if the delusion seems to be more strongly held than you would expect from your patient's circumstances and from your discussions with him about his delusion;
3. if the delusional belief is retained despite covering the appropriate areas of CBT that one would expect, theoretically, to be sufficient to have modified it.

If the underlying belief has not become apparent during therapy it may be difficult to uncover, either because the patient himself is unaware of it and/or because he has reason (e.g. shame) to hide it from you. One way of moving therapy along at this stage is for you to hypothesise about beliefs that could be relevant to the delusional belief and that the patient could hold, and then gently question your patient in an attempt to confirm or disconfirm your hypothesis. Once the underlying belief has been elicited it can then be treated like any other dysfunctional belief.

Example from clinical practice

Let us return to the patient described in Chapter 6, the middle-aged man who believed that two particular nurses on the ward wanted to put him in a coffin and cremate him alive. The reason he gave for this was that they knew about a crime he had committed some years ago. We were successful in modifying his beliefs about the crime, so that he accepted that this would not be a sufficient reason for anybody wanting to kill him, and we were able to show to his satisfaction that the two nurses concerned felt kindly towards him. He was able to use this information successfully to combat the fearful thoughts when they arose, but we were puzzled as to why the thoughts continued and why the CBT had not modified the underlying beliefs but only allowed them to be successfully countered when they occurred. We also wondered why these two particular nurses were seen as the potential killers, as other members of staff also knew of his prison record, but we were unable to come up with any convincing explanations. The patient did have a racial prejudice, but one nurse was black and one was white and the rest of the team was multiracial, so this did not seem to be a relevant underlying belief. Similarly, he did feel more confident with female staff, but one of the 'murderers' was female so his generally negative view of male staff did not seem to be relevant.

It was not until many months later, when another member of staff joined the ranks of potential murderers, that we suspected a previously undetected but very influential belief. A few days earlier the patient had hit the nurse badly enough for her to be off work for several days. He was adamant that he had not hit her because she had been trying to harm him in any way but because she would not give him his money out of hours so that he could go to buy cigarettes. If this incident was not a response to the delusion, could it have triggered it in some way, and if so, why? When asked if he thought the nurse would want to kill him because he had hit her, the patient looked slightly alarmed before admitting that he thought she might well do. This seemed to be a gross exaggeration of the nurse's likely reaction to the incident so we asked the patient why he thought the nurse would react in such an extreme way, what evidence did he have that people would respond to being assaulted by plotting murder? He was visibly agitated and discomforted by the questions but he was unable to come up with any supporting evidence or possible explanation as to why he made this assumption.

Reviewing what we knew about the patient, and bearing in mind his reaction to the questions, we came up with a possible hypothesis. We knew that the patient found it difficult to put himself in other people's positions and would assume that they felt exactly as he would in the same situation, so we postulated that perhaps the patient believed the nurse wanted to kill him because that is how he felt when people behaved aggressively towards him. If this hypothesis were true, the fact that the patient was not spontaneously admitting to it suggested that he might be ashamed of it, so we did some normalising/destigmatising work around automatic thoughts, noting that it was not uncommon to get aggressive and even violent thoughts towards people but that thinking and doing were quite different things. Having done this, we gently broached the question of how he felt towards people who were aggressive towards him, and in response to direct questioning he admitted that when this happened to him he would wish the other person was dead and sometimes even think about killing them.

Having elicited the patient's own response to these situations, and agreed that despite his thoughts, he never had and never would kill anyone, we then referred back to the nurse's reactions. We agreed that the nurse had probably felt pretty negative towards the patient and may well have wanted to hit him at the time, but noted that nevertheless she had not done so. We argued that as she had not hit him even in the heat of the moment, it would not be reasonable to suppose that she would attempt to retaliate more violently after the heat of the moment had faded.

We asked the patient why he had never killed anyone when the thought went through his mind and noted that it was because of the penalty that he would have to pay. (We took the opportunity of reinforcing the negative outcome, just in case the patient's own thoughts ever got more insistent.) We then looked at the penalty that the nurse would have to pay for harming the patient, namely loss of job, loss of profession, time in prison, separation from family, etc., to show that this would far outweigh any fleeting satisfaction she might receive from revenge.

Although we had normalised the occurrence of violent thoughts with the patient and shown why the nurse would not act in a violent manner towards the patient however she might feel, we were reluctant to leave the patient believing that the nurse did or had hated him so much as to want to kill him because of this incident. We noted that psychiatric nurses working on this particular ward must realise that there was a fair chance of being hit by a disturbed patient at some time or another and so the nurse concerned would not have asked to work on the ward if she felt so strongly about being hit that she would want to murder the patient later. It was suggested, therefore, that although it had no doubt been very unpleasant for the nurse to be hit and although she had no doubt felt fairly negative about the patient for a while afterwards, she would also be understanding about the incident, especially as the patient had since expressed his regret for his action. Having considered these other possible ways of viewing and reacting to the situation from the nurse's point of view, the patient felt able to check it out with the nurse concerned and she confirmed that the incident was now in the past as far as she was concerned and that she did not want to hurt the patient in any way for what had happened.

Subsequent enquiry revealed that the patient had hit the other two 'potential murderers' in the past, but so many years ago that the nurses themselves had to all intents and purposes forgotten about it. We were then able to use the same arguments as we had used with the third nurse to show that these two nurses would not be trying to kill the patient because they had been hit by him years before, and indeed that they did not even want to do so.

CBT WITH OTHER NON-PSYCHOTIC BELIEFS

CBT treats the person as a whole, not just his illness symptoms, so it may well be appropriate to undertake modification of dysfunctional beliefs that play no part in the delusions or hallucinations as such. For example, if the patient has low self-esteem because he has failed to achieve academic or occupational success, has no job, has no partner or family, etc. then it is appropriate to attempt to modify the underlying belief that these things indicate a person's worth.

Caution: When working with a patient who has had to drop out of education or who has failed to obtain employment at the expected level, a common mistake is to attempt to reassure him that of course he would have done well if it had not been for his illness, or that in the circumstances he is doing very well to attempt training for an unskilled job. The problem with this approach is that emphasising his previous academic achievements will covertly indicate to the patient that you, too, believe that academic success is important and to be sought after. Similarly, enthusiastically praising any occupational efforts will signal your views about the importance of job success. It is generally safer in such cases to adopt from the start an attitude of general indifference to educational achievement or occupational success, taking an approach that indicates that you value other factors, such as friendliness, generosity, independence, sense of humour, etc. as being the really important measures of a person's worth. This latter may be reinforced by asking the patient to describe what he likes about a particular friend and noting if, as is likely, worldly success is not one of the characteristics mentioned.

Modifying (challenging) the delusions

9

INTRODUCTION

Although the word 'challenge' is commonly used to describe this part of the therapy, where belief modification occurs, this work is rarely ever done as a direct challenge. It is probably more accurate to think of it as nibbling at the edges of the delusion, making little forays of attack and retreat to discover areas of vulnerability and the best strategies to use. The challenge may be directed at the delusional belief itself or at the factors that are underpinning and supporting it (see Appendix 2 for summary). As many different approaches as possible are used to build up the onslaught, until the delusion crumbles and modification becomes inevitable.

Logical reasoning and the gathering of evidence go hand in hand and are often used to support and progress each other as a particular line of argument is pursued. For example, in order for the patient to examine the evidence supporting his delusion he must feel that this is a worthwhile exercise to carry out. So before you can use the evidence collection and evaluation strategy, it may be necessary to use logical reasoning to cast a seed of doubt in the patient's mind about his belief, or at least to demonstrate to him that it is not unreasonable for other people to have some doubt about it. For example, a patient who visited our department became upset when he heard noises from the offices upstairs because he interpreted this as a sign that the people there were reading his mind. He would not consider looking for evidence to substantiate his belief because it was so obvious to him that it was true. It was only after the therapist had argued that it seemed to her that since the people upstairs had not seen him arrive (a fact that he readily accepted) they would not know to read his mind, even if they could do so, that he was prepared to discuss the evidence he had for mind reading. On other occasions, you may need the patient to recognise that there is some contradictory evidence to his delusional belief in order for him to tolerate the use of logical reasoning to question its plausibility. For example, a patient was so sure that he knew what people were going to say or do that he was not willing to entertain any doubts or questions about it, until he was faced with the disconfirming evidence of being hit by a fellow resident.

Although the development of alternative explanations is considered in this chapter as a separate strand of the challenging work, in practice it is closely tied up with the logical reasoning and evidence-gathering aspects of the work because the alternative explanation is both influenced by and in turn influences these other aspects. For example, in the case of the patient who believed that the noises from the rooms above indicated that the occupants were reading his mind, the therapist's immediate response was to express surprise on the grounds that she had assumed that the murmur of talking and scraping of chairs meant the same as they did on every other day of the week, namely that they were people in a meeting discussing some management issue about the wards. By expressing surprise and using the word 'assumed' for her own interpretation of events, the therapist was able to put forward an alternative explanation without implying that she disbelieved the patient's interpretation. This led naturally to a discussion about the patient's suggestion and hence to the first tentative piece of logical reasoning to question it. On the other hand, in the case of the patient who knew what people were going to do or say, it was not until after the evidence of his being hit had shown that this was not always true that we were able to make the first tentative suggestion that perhaps his ability to know when people were about to speak or leave the room could be based on his awareness of and sensitivity to social cues.

Although reality testing of at least some aspect of the delusional belief can occur quite early on in therapy (e.g. the patient who believed his thoughts were being spoken aloud was encouraged to ask people he trusted if they could hear this happening), it is more usual for it to occur in the later stages of therapy. One reason for this is that it must not occur until after the necessary insight and destigmatisation work has been done, and after the alternative explanations have been discussed, in order to ensure that the patient's interpretation of the results of the reality test will be non-delusional and in keeping with the overall goal of therapy. For some patients, reality testing may occur later rather than earlier in therapy because the patient may not see the point of testing out a belief he knows to be true or think that it is worth the effort involved to prove the obvious, so logical reasoning and evidence collection are often necessary in order to introduce an element of doubt in his mind. For others, where the delusion involves potential harm coming to the person, the patient may be unwilling to put his belief to the test if there is only an element of doubt in his mind; understandably, he will not want to risk a reality test until he is pretty certain that his belief is not true and therefore that the reality test is safe for him. For example, if a patient believes that if he cuts his hair something terrible will happen to him, the ultimate reality test of that belief would be for him to have his hair cut, but the arguments as to why no harm could befall him as a result of the haircut would need to be very persuasive to give him the courage and confidence to carry it out. In many cases, reality testing is the final conclusive part of therapy because the evidence it produces is unambiguous in its implications for that belief and so can have a powerful influence in bringing about or confirming the desired belief change.

MAKING THE GENERAL SPECIFIC

In the assessment interviews, some patients are very clear and direct in the delusional beliefs they report, for example 'Nurse Smith wants to put me in a coffin and burn me alive', whilst others are much vaguer, for example 'One of my family wants to harm me' or even just 'Someone wants to hurt me'. Your patient may be vague when talking to you about his delusions for a number of reasons other than the obvious one that the delusional belief itself is vague. For instance, your patient may find the subject matter unpleasant to think about and therefore want to avoid talking about it, or he may fear what would happen to himself or other people if he reveals what he knows. Other common reasons include thinking you will laugh about his delusion or not take it seriously, or thinking it will lead to an increase in his medication if the doctors come to hear about it. In some cases, the delusion may be such that not talking about it may be a direct consequence of the belief itself, e.g. if the patient believes he is a member of MI5, or it may just be that it is difficult to put into words because it involves feelings or concepts that are not covered by our everyday vocabulary. If your patient is reluctant to talk about his delusions or finds it difficult to put them into words then you should be gentle in your probing and not push him to give you more information than he is comfortable for you to have at that time, even if that means that you have to go cautiously, feeling your way with generalities rather than being able to work on specifics. In his role as 'patient', he may feel under a certain pressure to tell you personal things that he would rather keep quiet about, so you should be careful not to abuse your role as 'therapist' by persistent or intrusive questioning.

Where patients are willing to talk about their experiences and beliefs, you should ask questions along the lines 'who', 'what', 'when', 'where' and 'how' in order to obtain a more definite and precise description of the delusion. There are three main advantages for doing this as an early part of the CBT programme.

1. Specifics are usually easier to challenge than vague, general ideas so by clarifying the delusion this may open it up to rational arguments and reality tests that would not be possible with a vague idea. For example, it was possible to examine and test whether Nurse Smith wanted to put the patient in a coffin and have him cremated, but if the delusion had been framed as 'someone wants to kill me' then it would have been impossible to consider everybody in whatever area the 'someone' might have come from, or to consider every possible way that the patient might have been killed in order to prove that the delusion was not true.

2. Forcing the patient to think through the implications of his belief may constitute a challenge that actually weakens the belief. For example, one of our patients believed that someone on the ward was trying to stop him getting better, but when he considered each fellow patient in turn he dismissed each one as a possible culprit and thereby concluded that although he had this *feeling* about his fellow patients it could not be correct because no one of them would actually do such a thing.

3. If the patient is unable to make the general specific this may be used later on in therapy as evidence that the belief is founded on an intuition and not on real events. For example, it may be possible to argue along the lines that if the patient does not know *who* is trying to kill him then this suggests that no-one has done anything to indicate that he/she wants to do this and therefore that there is no objective evidence to back up the patient's general feeling.

As you ask the questions that cause your patient to think about his delusional belief in more detail, he may become aware of the inconsistencies in his responses or of gaps in his knowledge and realise what this implies, so you must question sensitively, backing off if he reacts adversely to any questions or is unable to answer. Because the vagueness of delusional beliefs may be useful as evidence that they are based on feelings rather than hard facts, you must be careful to accept the vagueness rather than forcing your patient to be more precise by your questioning. For example, you might summarise a vague belief that a family member is trying to cheat your patient along the lines of 'So you are sure that one of your family wants to take your money but you've really no idea at all which one that might be because none of them has ever given you any sign or indication that they are the one who wants to do this – is that right?'.

You should be particularly careful not to push your patient to resolve his vagueness with some alternative, delusional explanation that will be harder to modify than the original one. For example, in the case above, persistent questioning about who is trying to steal the patient's money might lead him to conclude that if it is not one of his family then it must be 'governmental powers'.

LOGICAL REASONING

For the most part, beliefs are only described as delusional because they are considered by other people to be unreasonable, so other people must have reasons for coming to this decision. Logical reasoning is a way of making use of these reasons in order to challenge the feasibility and truth of the delusion and hence to bring about its modification. It is almost certain that by the time you see your patient other people will already have told him that they do not believe his delusion to be true, but without effect, so the skill in using the logical reasoning approach is to develop a line of argument that moves in small steps and takes the patient inexorably from one step to another, so that the final step which challenges the delusion cannot be ignored or denied. An important part of this exercise is to establish each of the key steps of the argument *before* they are connected together, to ensure that they are not distorted by the delusion and that when the patient is exposed to the chain of logical reasoning he cannot 'escape' from it by changing his interpretation of any of the key steps.

Example from clinical practice

With the patient who feared being burnt alive by two nurses, one of the reasons why we believed this was delusional was that the nurses seemed to like him and therefore it would have been unreasonable that they would want to kill him in such an unpleasant fashion. The following line of argument was developed in order to establish that the nurses liked him and then to use this to challenge the delusional belief that they wanted to kill him.

'*Can someone who likes you also hate you?*' 'No'

'*Is Nurse Smith pleasant or unpleasant when he speaks to you?*' 'Pleasant'

'*Is Nurse Smith helpful or unhelpful when you've got a problem?*' 'Helpful'

'*If someone is pleasant and helpful to someone else is that a sign that they like them or a sign that they hate them?*' 'Like them'

'*You were telling me that Nurse Smith is pleasant and helpful to you, so is that a sign that he likes you or hates you?*' 'He likes me'

'How would someone feel about someone they wanted to burn alive; would they like them or hate them to want to do this?' 'Hate them'

'So would someone who likes someone, and doesn't hate them, want to burn them alive?' 'No'

'You know that Nurse Smith likes you because he's pleasant and helpful to you; and if he likes you he can't also hate you. But only someone who hated you would want to burn you alive. So it seems as if Nurse Smith can't want to burn you alive even though you get the feeling that he does; what do you think?' 'He can't want to, not really'

There are three key constituent parts or elements to this chain of logical reasoning leading up to the final step, namely (i) that you cannot both like and hate someone, (ii) that the nurses liked the patient and (iii) that only someone who hated the patient would want to burn him alive.

Deciding what lines of reason can be used

Although the lines of argument that can be developed will depend on the individual patient and his particular delusion, using logical reasoning to expose inconsistencies and contradictions in the belief is not as difficult as it might sound. First of all, you need to think about what lines of argument might be appropriate and then work out how each of these could be developed into a step-by-step logical sequence. A simple way of detecting possible lines of argument that you might be able to use is to ask yourself the question 'Why do *I* think the patient's delusion is not true?'. Your answer is likely to reveal at least some of the potential logical weaknesses and contradictions in your patient's belief.

Example from clinical practice

With the patient who feared he would be burnt alive by the two nurses, we were confident that this was a delusion because:

1. the nurses concerned did not dislike him;
2. even if they did dislike him, they did not dislike him enough to want to kill him;
3. even if they wanted to kill him, it would not be worth the penalty they would have to pay if caught;
4. it would be impossible for them to take a coffin up to the ward and force him into it against his will because he would fight back and other people would intervene;

5. it is not possible for someone to wander into a crematorium with a coffin and have it put into the furnace.

We have already seen how we used reasons (4) and (5) to lessen the distress caused by the thoughts, by showing that what the patient feared could not happen in practice (see p. 71). Any one of (1), (2) or (3) would be sufficient reason on its own why the nurses would not attempt to burn the patient alive but they represent different levels of liking/hating on the part of the nurses. The strongest reason for the nurses not wanting to kill him is that they like him and this is also probably the most pleasant belief for the patient to end up with, so it was the one that we wanted to prove and to use. However, if the patient had been convinced that the nurses disliked him then there would have been two possible courses of action. If the nurses did, in fact, like him then it should have been possible to prove that this was so, thereby changing the patient's belief about the nurses liking him: once this new belief was established it could be used to counter the delusional belief in the way described above. However, if the nurses did not, in fact, like the patient, then we would have had to resort to reason (2), namely that there is a difference between disliking someone and wanting to kill them. If we had been unable to establish this latter fact to the patient's satisfaction then we would have had to resort to reason (3), that even if the nurses had wanted to kill him it would not have been worth the penalty they would have had to pay if caught. Again, it would have been necessary to get the patient's whole-hearted agreement to this latter fact before it could have been used to counter the delusion.

Although theoretically speaking it was only necessary to show that the nurses liked the patient in order to disprove his delusion, in practice we used the other lines of reason as well because usually the more lines of argument and evidence you can amass against a delusion, the more likely it is to shift. However, when discussing reasons (2) and (3) we had to be careful not to imply that we were considering them because perhaps the nurses might not like him after all. In order to avoid this risk we prefaced our logical arguments with a confirmation of the desired belief, e.g. 'We know that the nurses like you and so wouldn't want to harm you in any way, but even if someone did dislike someone...' or '... even if someone did hate someone enough to want to kill them...' etc.

Related to the question 'Why do I think the belief is a delusion?' is the question 'If this delusion were true in fact, what would follow from that? What would be different from how things actually are?'. Thinking about the implications of the delusion in this way may expose inconsistencies in the belief or contradictions between the belief and reality. For example, a patient believed that his next-door neighbour had magical powers and could see into the future. But if this were true the neighbour would have been able to see the winning lottery prize numbers and become a millionaire and would not be living in the run-down council house next door to the patient. In the case of the patient who thought he was going to be burnt alive, if his belief had been true this would have meant that the nurses concerned were potential murderers, and if that were true then we might have expected to have had some indication of this from their characters or behaviour, but there was none. As with all logical reasoning, these lines of argument can only be used to challenge the delusional belief if the patient agrees with each of the key steps. For example, in the first of the above two cases the patient would have to agree that a millionaire would not continue to live in his old council house, and in the second case the patient would have to agree that potential murderers do not behave entirely like ordinary people.

Deciding what lines of reason are most suitable to use

As we saw in the clinical examples above, you cannot use a particular line of argument to contradict a delusional belief unless your patient agrees with all the steps in it. So, having identified a potential line of logical reasoning you must find out what your patient thinks or believes about each of the key steps. Suppose, for example, that a patient believes he has ants living under his skin. A potential line of argument to counter this belief is that ants need to breathe oxygen in order to live and there is no oxygen under the skin. But this argument will only be effective if the patient agrees both that ants need oxygen to live and that there is no oxygen under the skin, so you would have to find out if he knows that insects have to breathe air and what he understands about the construction of a human limb.

The more secure the constituent parts of the argument, the less likely it is that the chain of logical reasoning will be rejected or distorted when its conclusion is set against the contradictory delusional belief. Knowledge and beliefs that the patient already holds are the most secure against change, so wherever possible you would try to use lines of argument that rely on already accepted points. Where the patient does not have the necessary knowledge this can be provided for him as part of the therapy, and providing it is compatible with his existing beliefs and knowledge about the world, it is only slightly less secure against change than pre-existing knowledge. Where the patient holds an inaccurate belief or has incorrect knowledge about a key element of the argument then it may be possible to change this during therapy, but beliefs that have had to be modified or knowledge that has had to be corrected is much less likely to stand firm against the delusion and so would only be used if more effective lines of argument were not available, or as an extra line once the delusion had been seriously undermined. For example, in the case above, if the patient was a biology student and already knew that all living things need oxygen to live and that the skin on an arm is firmly attached to the flesh underneath, then this line of argument would be difficult for him to dispute. If, on the other hand, he knew little about biology then it would be possible to explain to him why all living things, including insects, need to breathe to live and why living skin must be attached firmly to the underlying flesh. If, however, he was already sure that there was a layer of air between skin and flesh then it might be possible to correct this belief by discussion and/or consulting textbooks, but when confronted with the complete line of argument against his delusion he is likely to 'realise' that he must have been correct after all to believe that the skin is not joined to the flesh.

In order to decide what line of reason to pursue and to assess whether the patient already believes the constituent parts, you should put the relevant questions to your patient in a neutral, conversational way, as part of one of your general discussions. In this way your patient is less likely to be aware of the implications of his answers for his delusional belief. You should be careful not to ask any direct questions that could challenge the delusion too soon as this may lead to other parts of the argument being distorted before they can be strengthened (see section below). For example, in the case just mentioned, the patient is unlikely to have considered the question of how the ants breathe so asking this question baldly might force him to reason that they must be breathing air from under his skin, thereby establishing a dysfunctional belief that will effectively undermine that particular line of argument.

Strengthening the constituent parts of the argument

The purpose of developing a step-by-step argument against a delusion, of showing your patient that his delusional belief is not compatible with some other established fact, is that your patient will then change his delusional belief. The last thing you want, therefore, is for your patient to change his interpretation of the established fact so that it becomes consistent with the delusion. We know that strongly held beliefs can have considerable power in distorting the interpretation of evidence and reason, even to the point of completely reversing the interpretation of contradictory evidence, so it is essential that when the inconsistency is exposed the contradictory, non-delusional parts are so strong that they cannot be re-evaluated in line with the delusion. Therefore, once you have established that there is a line of argument to contradict the delusion, you must strengthen the non-delusional part before you attempt to use it against the delusion. For example, the patient who believes he has insects under his skin might agree that ants need to breathe to live and agree that there is no air under his skin, but before these two facts are linked together to counter the delusional belief the therapist should strengthen them by explaining why ants could not possibly live without oxygen and why it is impossible for living skin to be separated from the flesh beneath. Similarly with the patient who feared being burnt alive, we took great care to strengthen the patient's belief that the nurses liked him, by gathering so much supporting evidence that this fact could not be disputed or re-evaluated.

When seeking to establish and strengthen the constituent parts of the logical argument, it may be necessary to establish the required facts about people or things in general before attempting to establish the same facts as they affect the patient. Questions relating to other people and their situations are less likely to be perceived as being relevant to the patient's situation and therefore are less likely to be distorted by the delusional belief and perceived as a challenge to it. In the chain of logical reasoning detailed on pp. 123–4 the essential parts of the logical argument were established first in terms of a general 'someone'. Similarly, with the man who fears he has ants living under his skin, the reason why ants have to have oxygen to live would be established first in terms of living things in general and only when that belief is secure should this be extended to ants in particular, because as soon as ants are mentioned the patient is likely to make a connection with his delusional belief.

The constituent elements of the argument will be more secure against subsequent change if they are supported and strengthened by evidence that is easy to confirm and that is not open to alternative interpretations. For this reason, objective evidence obtained from events and situations is preferable to evidence based on subjective factors such as attitudes and feelings. For example, the evidence collected to support the conclusion that the nurses liked the patient concentrated on actual incidents where the nurses had said or done pleasant things for him, incidents which were recorded so that the patient's memory of them could not be distorted subsequently. If we had relied on smiles or pleasant tones of voice, these would have been easier to re-evaluate when set against the delusion (e.g. 'I thought he had smiled at me but now I think it was more of a sly smirk').

Using the logical argument to make the contradictions explicit

Because it is so important to strengthen the constituent parts of the logical argument before it is used to counter the delusional belief, it is usual to ask the initial questions and to work on establishing the constituent parts at times that are well separated from any discussion you may have about the delusional belief itself. Ideally you would do this work in separate sessions, but if you are pressed for time and want to use a single session then you should ensure that something else is discussed in between; certainly you should not move immediately from discussing the delusion to discussing the things that are going to be used in the argument against it, or move immediately between key elements of the argument. Even with this precaution, your patient may see the implication of your work on the different parts of arguments, especially if you seem to be pushing something too enthusiastically, so if you suspect that your patient is beginning to make the connections himself, too soon, you should back off rapidly and turn to another topic of conversation. Otherwise, as we have seen, you run the risk of having the non-delusional parts of the argument distorted to fit in with the delusion, and then you will not be able to use that particular line of logical reasoning to challenge the delusion.

Before you expose the chain of logical reasoning to your patient, you should think ahead as to whether there is any other way that he might resolve the apparent contradiction other than realising that his delusional belief seems to be in error. If other possible resolutions do exist then you should remove them or effectively counter them before you expose the logical argument. For example, in the case of the patient who believes he has ants under his skin, there is the potential risk that, when faced with the logical argument that contradicts his delusion, he might conclude that although the ants need oxygen to live they are getting it from his blood-stream or that although the skin is normally attached to the flesh underneath in his case the ants have eaten away a space in between which is now filled with air. In order to ensure that he does not come to either of these conclusions, the therapist would need to establish (i) that only specially adapted water creatures can get oxygen from a liquid, that all land creatures, including ants, need to get oxygen in a gaseous form, and (ii) that skin cannot live if cut from the flesh beneath and that one way of testing whether the skin is living or not is to see if it can feel a pinprick. Of course, there will be occasions when your patient will use an escape route that you have not anticipated. For example, in the case above, when faced with the apparent conflict between the established facts of the argument and his strongly held delusion, the patient might conclude that the ants are not ordinary ants but a special sort of swimming ant, previously unknown to science, that can get its oxygen from liquids like blood. If this happens then you have to challenge the escape route in the same way that you would challenge any other delusional idea or belief. The reason for trying to anticipate the possible escape routes and to close them off is that it is easier to establish a belief about something that is neutral for the patient than it is to challenge a conclusion that he has already come to, especially if that conclusion enables him to make sense of and to reconcile the apparent contradiction to his delusional belief.

When you have decided that the time is right to expose the logical argument to your patient, you should consider how to do this in a way that will not be experienced by him as you triumphantly proving him wrong. I find it can be helpful to introduce the subject by saying that I have been thinking about what the patient has told me in previous sessions and noticed something that was a bit puzzling, or that did not seem to quite make sense, and that I would like his views on it. Going over what he has told me previously gives me the opportunity to reinforce the non-delusional components of the argument as the chain of logical reasoning is developed. For example, I might say something like 'I've been thinking about what you were telling me last week and something has struck me as a bit strange. You were saying that Nurse Smith and Nurse Brown are always pleasant and helpful when they see you or when you ask for something and that that was a good sign that they must like you – and I am sure you are absolutely right in that because people don't do nice things for people if they dislike them. And then I thought about something you were saying the other day, that someone would only want to burn someone alive if they really hated them – and that's certainly true. So it occurred to me that as Nurse Smith and Nurse Brown so obviously like you, then they can't hate you, and this would mean that they can't really want to burn you alive after all. Does that make sense? What do you think?'.

In order to make it easier for the patient to change his delusional belief, and in order to guide this change in the right direction, it is often helpful at this stage to bring in the alternative view. For example, in the case just mentioned, having made the argument explicit I then went on to add 'Although the thoughts about the nurses seem to be true when they occur, I wondered if they could be like the automatic thoughts we were discussing the other day, which can make people *feel* very frightened even though they're not actually true in fact – is that possible?'.

Note that when you present the line of logical reasoning in this way it is usual to go through only the key elements of the argument and not all the steps that were needed to establish them. However, if the patient should question the truth of the key elements then you can remind him of the steps you went through previously to show that they were true.

Summary of how to develop and use logical reasoning

1. What potential arguments against the delusion exist from your point of view?
2. What are the patient's views/beliefs about the constituent parts of the argument?
3. If the patient has existing beliefs about the constituent parts that are accurate, strengthen them.

4. If the patient has no existing belief/knowledge about a constituent part, establish the appropriate belief/knowledge and strengthen it.
5. If the patient has an existing belief/knowledge about the constituent part that is inaccurate, attempt to modify it and then strengthen the new, accurate belief/knowledge.
6. Consider whether there are any ways that the patient could resolve the apparent contradiction between the line of argument and his delusion other than by modifying the delusional belief. If there are possible escape routes, seal them off.
7. Present the argument, summarising the reason and evidence in favour of the non-delusional, constituent part as you do so.
8. Support the alternative belief that replaces the delusion.

Example from clinical practice

A patient suddenly developed the unpleasant belief that there were little men in his head, based on the sensation of feet pattering from one side of his head to the other. This sensation seemed to be a mixture of touch and sound. He accepted that he had schizophrenia and knew from earlier therapy that this could produce some strange hallucinatory experiences, so it was not necessary to do any preparatory work to ensure that the alternative belief, namely that these sensations were caused by his illness, would be acceptable to him.

I asked myself why I did not believe as my patient did and came up with a number of reasons including (i) that my patient had a brain in his head and therefore could not have a cavern there as well and (ii) that the little men could not have got into his head without leaving a hole around the entry point.

I decided to develop these two lines of reasoning into watertight, logical arguments and then, if they were sufficient to modify his delusional belief, to support this modification by discussing my other reasons with him. Remember that the answers to the questions detailed below would have been obtained at different times before they were brought together into the two chains of logical reasoning.

How do you know the little men are in your head? How long have they been there?
I can hear them and feel them running from one ear to the other; they're in a large cavern, I can hear the echoes. They've been there a couple of days, since Sunday night.

How many of them are there?
About half a dozen, I think.

How big are they?
About one and a half inches high and half an inch wide.

How big is the cavern?
About seven inches by four inches.

How did they get into the cavern?
Through my ears – they can't have got in anywhere else because, as my friend pointed out, there are no scars on my face.

These questions produced the basic information required to indicate where the contradictions lay. It was important to establish the physical size of the cavern and the little men because it would have been unhelpful if, when faced with the argument that he must have a brain in his head and so there could be no room for the little men as well, the patient had retreated to the position of a tiny cavern and tiny men, as these latter would have been harder to disprove than the patient's original perception. It was agreed, therefore, that the men were 1½″ tall, and that the cavern must be at least 6″ wide and at least 2″ tall for most of the distance across.

The contradictions to be used were based on the solid physical properties of the little men and the cavern in which they were running, so it would have been unhelpful if the patient were to resolve the contradictions by modifying the delusion from physical to spiritual or ghostly men, as such entities might well be able to move through brain tissue. In order to prevent this modification from occurring it was established and agreed at an early stage that if the patient could hear and feel the men this must mean that they were physical, solid objects of some sort.

The next set of questions was used to establish that the patient could not have a cavern in his head as well as a normal, functioning brain. The patient had studied A level human biology and so knew about the brain and how it worked and so was able to answer the questions appropriately, but had he not done so we would have had to establish the facts first, using a biology book and/or medical colleagues as the authority on these matters. We could not have proceeded with this line of reasoning unless and until the patient had accepted the basic, biological facts about the brain being responsible for sight, hearing and speech.

Why do people have heads?
To hold their brains.

How big is the brain?
Almost the same size as your skull.

So normally the brain fills the person's head, with no gaps?
Yes.

What does the brain do?
It sees, hears and makes you talk.

So if someone can see, hear and talk normally does that mean their brain is normal?
Yes.

Can the brain ever get squashed up?
Yes, if there's a tumour.

Does a squashed-up brain work normally?
No.

Would it affect the way the person sees, hears and talks if his brain was squashed up?
Yes.

Can you see, hear and talk?
Yes.

So if you can see, hear and talk normally does that mean you have a normal brain?
Yes.

So if you have a normal brain, that's not squashed up, how can there be a big 7" by 4" cavern in your head?
I suppose there can't be.

In establishing that the patient had a perfectly normal brain we used functions that there could be no doubt about his being able to do. The patient had complained earlier that his thoughts felt a bit muddled so we were careful not to use thinking as an indication of normal brain physiology.

The next line of reasoning was used to add weight to the conclusion from the previous logical reasoning exercise and was set to establish that the men could not have entered his head through his ears without damaging his ears so badly that he would not be able to hear.

When I learnt biology I was taught that the passage in the ear led to an eardrum, did you cover that in your course?
Yes.

What does the eardrum do?
It vibrates to sounds and this is turned into nerve signals that get sent to the brain.

So it can't do that if it is damaged at all?
No.

How do you know the little men didn't get in through your face?
Because it would have left a scar at least half an inch across,
probably more, so I would have been able to see it.

*So if they had got in through your ears they would have made a
hole at least half an inch across in your eardrum, too?*
Yes.

*So you would not be able to hear through that ear with a hole that
size?*
No, that's right.

Can you hear with both ears at the moment?
Yes.

*So you can't have a hole in either of your eardrums and so the men
couldn't have got in that way?*
No, I suppose not.

*And you know they can't have got in any other way because there
are no scars on your head. And I guess there would have been quite
a lot of blood around on your pillow on Monday morning if
something as large as 1½" × ½" had forced its way through your
skin?*
Yes, that's true.

*So no little men can have got into your head? There can't be any
little men in your head?*
No.

*So it sounds as if the **feelings** you get of tiny pattering feet running
across your head must be another example of your brain halluci-
nating, but this time through the sense of touch as well as sound.
What do you think? It must be a horrible feeling, but I suppose at
least it's reassuring to know that there aren't really creatures living
in your head and that your brain is still perfectly OK.*

These two arguments were sufficiently robust that when they contradicted the delusional belief it was the delusional belief and not some
element of the arguments that was changed.

Note: The series of questions given for the above patient represents the
course of the logical arguments pursued to expose the contradictions. In
practice, you would never fire a series of questions at a patient in this
way, the logical argument would be developed in a natural way during
one or more discussions. Nor would you necessarily need to use all the

questions in the series in order to develop the argument; depending on the strength of the patient's delusional and other beliefs about the world, he may readily move through several steps in one jump. You certainly do not want to bore or appear to patronise your patient by asking him a lot of 'obvious' questions, but equally you must be careful not to assume that what seems obvious to you is obvious to him. The delusional belief can have a powerful, distorting effect on the way the patient perceives and understands things. For example, with the patient above, it may seem silly to ask why people have heads and what the head contains, because within our own belief system it is perfectly obvious what is there: however, for the patient who believed he had a large cavern in his head it was not at all 'obvious' that he had a brain and therefore this had to be established. The stronger the delusional belief, the more meticulous you have to be to go step by step to make the argument watertight so that it cannot be disputed when it is set against the delusion.

EVIDENCE FOR AND AGAINST

You need to ask your patient questions about his delusional beliefs in order to build up an accurate picture of what each belief might be based on and what evidence he has to support it, because you cannot target and undermine something that you are not aware of. The evidence you need to collect is evidence from the past, evidence that occurs during the course of therapy and evidence that is produced from reality testing. The evidence that your patient recalls from the past is likely to be biased in favour of the delusion because, like any other strongly held belief, the delusional belief will not only have distorted the way that events were interpreted, but will also have biased the attention he paid to them, i.e. he will have selectively attended to evidence that confirmed his belief whilst tending to ignore any evidence that contradicted it. Nevertheless, when talking to your patient you should be on constant alert for anything he tells you that might run contrary to his delusional belief. If he gives you this evidence freely, in the early stages of therapy, then it is likely that he does not appreciate the contradiction, so you should be careful not to point it out to him but just make a note of it for later consideration and use.

In some cases it is relatively easy, at least in principle, to see what evidence would be needed to disprove the delusion, for example, with the patient who believed he owned houses in Kent and Cornwall or with the patient who believed that the water was poisoned with arsenic. In other cases, however, it may be difficult to see what evidence could disprove the delusion in the form it takes, for example the patient who believed his son intended to poison him in order to inherit his money or the patient who believed that God would be angry if she stopped fasting. In these latter cases, where it is difficult to collect evidence directly related to the delusion itself, it may be possible to collect evidence about some implication of the delusion, i.e. about something that would necessarily follow if the delusion were true. The line of argument for this approach is 'If the delusion is true, then X must follow, so if X is not true then the delusion cannot be true either'. For example, in the case above, the only way of directly testing whether the patient's son intended to poison him or not would be to ask the son; but the patient is unlikely to be convinced by his denial. However, the implications of this delusion, namely that his son does not love or care for him, that the patient has enough money to make murder worthwhile and that the son would be prepared to risk prison and losing everything for the sake of the money, are potentially more easy to contradict. As a general principle, whilst it is possible to collect evidence about present situations, no direct evidence can exist about future events. In the second example given above, there is no direct way of determining whether God would be angry or not if the patient stopped her fast because there is absolutely no way of checking out how God might feel about something. However, one of the implications of this delusional belief is that God requires people in hospital to starve themselves, for no apparent reason, so you might be able to counter this implication by seeking the views of the acknowledged experts from the patient's own religious group.

Is the delusion based on a strong feeling but little evidence?

As we saw earlier in this chapter (p. 122) some patients are not able to produce any evidence to substantiate their delusion – they just know it is so and that is that. For example, one of our patients just knew that his father had been replaced by a double who looked and behaved exactly the same as his real father. Paradoxically, it may be the very strength of conviction in the delusion that accounts for the lack of evidence to support it, as the patient has never felt the need to find any. If this is the case with your patient, be careful not to force him to come up with some supporting evidence by your persistent questioning. It may even be appropriate to note that the belief is built on an inner certainty that does not require any evidence to back it up, for example, 'You know that your father is not really your father, that he was replaced by an identical double three years ago, and it's so obvious that you've never needed to have any evidence to confirm that that's so, is that right?'.

Where a delusion is based on a very strong feeling of certainty that is not backed up by objective evidence, the approach to modification is to promote the patient's understanding that a feeling, however persuasive, does not necessarily guarantee that it is true, and then to go on to examine the accuracy of this particular (delusional) feeling. Wherever possible, evidence that is inconsistent with or that contradicts the delusion is collected, either from everyday events or from targeted reality testing. For example, in the above case, the evidence collected about the patient's father might include statements from close family members and observation of how the father behaves, or it might involve the patient questioning his father about memories of his childhood that the patient could then check for accuracy. The contradictory evidence collected is then used with any appropriate logical reasoning to show that the delusional belief must be wrong despite the feeling of certainty. Depending on the delusion, it may be possible to prove only that the delusion is wrong some of the time, not that it is always or even usually wrong, but where the delusion is based solely on the feeling then this is enough. If the feeling of certainty can be shown to be misleading/wrong at least some of the time, then the feeling of certainty is not and cannot be a reliable indicator of the truth and hence there is no reliable evidence that the delusional belief is true.

Is the evidence given in support of the delusion based on someone else's interpretations and beliefs?

As we have seen throughout this book, there is no clear distinction between a psychotic and a non-psychotic belief and certainly some non-psychotic people can hold some very strange beliefs and interpret things in some very strange ways. This is particularly likely to occur in the realm of the occult and paranormal. Where these strange beliefs and interpretations are compatible with the patient's delusion then he may seize upon them as evidence to support his delusion. In this case, the only way of undermining this support is to challenge these other beliefs and interpretations.

If you know exactly where these other beliefs have come from then this gives you a much better chance of successfully challenging them. So if your patient supports his delusion by quoting a book or referring to a film, then you should make every effort to read the book or see the film. It is not impossible that your patient has misconstrued what he read or saw, in which case you will be able to discuss this misunderstanding with him, but if he is accurate in his understanding then reading the book may enable you not only to challenge the particular views it contains but also to use other arguments to discredit the authority of the author. For example, one of our patients refused to take his medication because he had read a book that ascribed the symptoms of schizophrenia to an emerging spirituality whose progress was halted by medication, so it was the fault of the medication that the sufferer remained in this disturbed, semi-spiritual state. Having read the book, I was able to point out that people had suffered from schizophrenia before medication was available and furthermore that the old mental hospitals had been full of people with unremitted schizophrenia despite their having no medication, so clearly medication was not to blame for their failing to get better or to progress spiritually to a peaceful, enlightened state. There were also several other weaknesses in the author's argument that were easy to criticise once I knew of them.

It may seem a daunting task, having to read through some rather strange book or see some way-out fantasy film in order to discredit a delusion, but it certainly broadens one's horizons!

Is the evidence given in support of the delusion a distortion of something that really happened?

Often the evidence that a patient gives in support of his delusional belief is true in that the event or situation described did actually happen, but it is untrue in that the interpretation of what happened has been distorted. For example, one piece of evidence that a patient gave to support her belief that her neighbours were plotting against her was that they called in the council officials to visit her. It was true that a couple of council workers had visited and insisted on entering her flat, but only because there was a steady drip of water from her bathroom floor through to the neighbours' flat beneath and she had refused to answer the neighbours when they had called to tell her about it. The misinterpretation of evidence may be the result of the distorting effect of the delusion itself, as in the case just mentioned, or it may be the result of biases in the way the patient thinks, the so-called errors of thinking that were mentioned briefly in Chapter 1 (p. 13). Whatever the cause, the misinterpretation must be challenged and corrected in order to be able to remove what is seen by the patient as evidence that proves his delusion to be true.

If the evidence has been distorted because of the influence of the delusion, then the usual way of attempting to modify this is to use alternative explanations/interpretations to counter the distorted interpretation (see next section). This may be backed up by logical reasoning, evidence collection and reality testing, as appropriate. For example, in the case just described, the alternative explanation you would go for would be that the neighbours called in the council because they were worried about their ceiling and carpets getting soaked. You would aim to establish with the patient that there was water leaking from her bathroom into the neighbours' flat below and that the neighbours had tried to contact her about it but she had not opened the door to them. You might then be able to reason along the lines of what, in these circumstances, someone ought to do. By agreeing what would be reasonable behaviour from the neighbours in these circumstances, you would be able to suggest that it was at least possible that they had only called in the council in order to get the leak stopped, and therefore that this action of itself did not necessarily indicate that they were plotting against her.

If the evidence has been distorted by an error or bias in thinking, the approach to modifying the misinterpretation is essentially the same as if the distortion is caused by the delusion, but if the patient recognises that he is inclined to make this type of thinking error then you can use this insight to cast more doubt on his interpretation. For example, with one of our patients who interpreted a salesgirl's glance to mean that she thought he was ugly, we made a suggestion along the lines 'We've noticed that you tend to think things involve you or are related to you when they are not, especially where young women are concerned, so I wonder if, when you interpreted the salesgirl's look as a sign that she thought you were ugly, that could have been another example of you doing that? ... because from what you were telling me, there doesn't seem to be any other evidence to support that she might have been thinking about you in a critical way'.

Is the evidence given in support of the delusion itself delusional?

It is not uncommon for other delusions or delusional misinterpretations to be given as evidence in support of the delusion; for example, one of our patients knew that a fellow patient wanted to take over his body because the newscaster on TV the evening before had warned him about it. Where this occurs you have to modify the supporting delusion even if that delusion is harmless in itself, in order to remove the piece of evidence that is supporting the delusion you do want to change. In the case just mentioned, this would mean tackling the delusional belief about the newscaster talking directly to the patient, before you could show that this was not valid evidence to support the delusion about the patient taking over his body. Having to sidetrack in this way to tackle other delusional beliefs can be time consuming, because even though they may not be troublesome in themselves, these other delusional beliefs can also be firmly held and so difficult to shift. You may even be unlucky enough to find that they in their turn are supported by yet other delusional beliefs, in which case you may have no option but to sidetrack yet again to modify these other delusions. If the evidence provided by the supporting delusional belief is fairly insignificant in the overall picture for the troublesome delusion then you may be able to leave it and hope that the other evidence that is collected and the logical reasons that can be produced are so strong that they outweigh this one piece of evidence and the delusional belief can be modified anyway. However, if the delusional evidence is a significant piece of support for the targeted delusion then you may have no option but to try to undermine it by modifying the supporting delusions.

Collect evidence to contradict the delusion

Ideally, the evidence you collect and build up concerning the delusional belief directly contradicts or at least is inconsistent with it, and ideally you would want to collect as much evidence as possible, as there seems to be something persuasive about sheer quantity of evidence when it is amassed together. But whereas you can ask your patient directly for the evidence he has that confirms his belief (e.g. 'How do you know that...') in most cases it would be unproductive to ask a similar direct question about disconfirming evidence (e.g. 'Do you have any reasons for believing that ... is not true?'), because if your patient was aware it contradicted his belief then he would either have modified his interpretation of it so that it was no longer contradictory or he would have modified his delusional belief to accommodate it. Furthermore, as we noted when considering how to approach questioning patients about their delusions, any direct question that implies that you doubt your patient's version of events is likely to lead to loss of rapport and to adversely affect your therapeutic alliance. For these reasons, when collecting evidence to use against the delusional belief, you will have to elicit most of this information from your patient by asking him specific rather than general questions.

A useful guide as to what specific questions might be appropriate for this purpose is to ask yourself the questions 'What would it be like if the delusion were true? How would things be different?' because the answers may direct you to areas of potential relevance. For example, in the case of the patient who believed his father had been replaced by a double, if the delusion were true then this would mean, amongst other things, that the double would not have any memories of the patient's childhood except what he had learnt from other people. Thus you might ask your patient 'Does your father's double ever talk about when you were a child? What has he talked about?' etc. The information is just noted at this stage.

Exposing the patient to the contradictory evidence

When asking questions to elicit evidence against the delusion you should be careful to do it in such a way as to not expose your patient to the contradiction at too early a stage. As with logical reasoning, if a piece of contradictory evidence is brought to the patient's attention too soon it may not be secure enough to stand against the delusion and therefore may be reinterpreted in a way that is compatible with the delusion. Therefore, as with logical reasoning, where contradictory evidence exists you may need to support and firmly establish the contradictory aspect of the evidence before using it to challenge the delusional belief, to ensure that when the challenge is made the contradictory evidence cannot be explained away.

Another (though less likely) risk of bringing a piece of contradictory evidence to the patient's attention too soon is that the delusion will be adapted to incorporate the apparently contradictory evidence, which is undesirable if it is adapted in a way that will make it harder to disprove. Therefore it may be appropriate to agree the specifics of the patient's delusional belief before doing the work to challenge it. For example, in the case of the patient who believed he had little men in his head, the fact that the cavern was large and filled with air was noted before the lines of argument were set against the delusion, to make it harder for the patient to subsequently change his delusion to tiny men living in the ventricles or blood vessels.

In order to avoid revealing the contradictory evidence too soon, you may have to ask the questions about the potentially disconfirming evidence at a different time or in a different session from questions directly related to the delusional belief; for example, in the case where the patient's delusional belief about being taken over by a fellow patient was supported by the warning from the newscaster, you would not ask the patient whether or not the newscaster knew him personally immediately after talking about the personal information the newscaster had given him. Neither should you attempt to elicit too many pieces of contradictory evidence at one time; if your patient is very sensitive about having his delusion doubted then you might have to separate all of these questions by general conversation about neutral or unrelated issues.

However careful you are to separate your questions about the contradictory evidence, your patient may make the connection between the information you are asking about and his delusional belief and become suddenly aware of the contradiction; the signs to look out for are if he appears suddenly puzzled or disconcerted or becomes suspicious, or if he makes some reference to the delusion itself. If this occurs at an early stage, before it is safe to expose the contradiction, you should back off rapidly by showing little interest in his answer and by changing the topic or the direction of the conversation.

When you consider the contradictory evidence is secure against reinterpretation, and the patient has been otherwise prepared for the belief modification, you may gently introduce the contradiction as a 'challenge' to the delusion.

This may be done by asking your patient the appropriate questions close together, so that he becomes aware of the contradiction for himself and has to make an adjustment in his delusional belief accordingly. Alternatively, you may 'float' the contradiction past your patient. For example, in the case of the patient who believed his father was a double you might float one of the inconsistencies thus: 'I've been thinking about what you've told me about your real father and about his double. You were telling me a couple of weeks ago that the double had been talking at dinner about an incident that happened with your real father when you were on a fishing trip together, how he had given you a can of beer and made you promise not to tell your mother because you were only eight and she would have been very cross with him – do you remember? And both of you must have kept that secret because it was the first time that your mother had ever heard the tale? Well, it occurred to me that only your real father could have known of this incident, because it was a secret between the two of you, so it seems strange that the double could have talked about it...'. The advantage of floating ideas past your patient rather than making the contradictions explicit through your questions is that it gives you better control over how thoroughly or sharply you expose the contradictions, and also enables you to support the contradictory part in order to protect it against reinterpretation. Furthermore, it may give you the opportunity to see how he is going to react to it; if it looks as if his reaction is not going to be favourable you can back off, without losing or weakening the contradictory evidence by forcing your patient to re-evaluate it in line with his delusion. If there appears to be no shift in the delusional belief when the contradictory evidence is exposed then it is better to withdraw rapidly to a position of puzzlement, reinforcing the desired part of the contradiction as you do so; for example, 'It's a bit puzzling, that, isn't it, because the double can't possibly have learnt about that incident from anyone and yet somehow he was able to talk about it. Oh well, it's not important, what I really wanted to talk to you about is...'.

Weighing up the evidence 'for' and 'against'

Once your patient has agreed that it is possible that his belief may not be entirely correct, for example as the result of logical reasoning or a particularly impressive piece of evidence, then it may be appropriate to engage in evidence collection in a more formal fashion, as a prelude to a formal evaluation of the evidence. The evidence your patient collects may be 'for' and 'against' either the delusional belief or the alternative belief. The evidence used in both these exercises is essentially the same, but since most people find it pleasanter to prove that they are right about something than to discover that they have been wrong, where the alternative belief is incompatible with the delusional belief and your patient is prepared to consider it as a possibility, then it is preferable to check out this alternative belief rather than the delusional one.

The evidence collected by your patient may come from his past experience or may be collected during the course of therapy. Your aim is to discredit any evidence given in favour of the delusion so that your patient no longer sees it as supporting the delusion, or at least to weaken its significance by casting doubt on it or by minimising its importance. At the same time, your aim is to build up the evidence against the delusional belief and in favour of the alternative belief.

When collecting evidence around the delusional belief, it is often helpful to have an agreement with your patient that only solid, objective evidence that would be acceptable in a court of law is permissible. For example, you would accept that the patient has a 'feeling' that something is so but not that this feeling is hard evidence, because unsubstantiated feelings or intuitions are not accepted in courts of law. (This would also provide you with the opportunity to discuss why feelings are not acceptable in a court of law, namely because they are known to be unreliable and misleading.)

Needless to say, you do not need to cast the same critical eye over the evidence that your patient gives you against his delusional belief as you would over evidence given in support, and nor do you need to point out its inadequacies. Nevertheless, although you would accept without challenge any evidence that your patient produced against his delusional belief, it is better not to stress any inappropriate evidence since he may later come to reject it himself. For example, one of our patients argued that she could not be subnormal because she was able to look after her personal hygiene. We accepted this piece of evidence, refraining from pointing out that subnormal people can have perfectly good personal hygiene, but we took care to find more solid evidence to support her conclusion, not least because there was the risk that in the future she would meet someone with learning difficulties who was clean and well presented (see p. 195 for details).

You should not embark on a formal weighing up of the evidence unless and until you are sure that the outcome will be favourable because you do not want to risk strengthening the delusion by confirming that there is more evidence in favour of it than against it. Ideally, you would not proceed with a formal weighing up of the evidence until you had eliminated every piece of the evidence supporting the delusion, but if that is not possible you should have a good idea from your discussions with your patient about the individual bits of evidence that he will produce and how much weight he puts on each of them.

To help your patient weigh up the evidence it may be formally written on a sheet of paper, divided into two columns headed evidence 'for' and 'against'. You may assist your patient, if he so wishes, by summarising the evidence and writing it down for him whilst he is thinking about it, but once you engage on the formal weighing up exercise it is important that you are not seen to be partisan with respect to the evidence that goes into it and that you allow your patient to come to his own conclusions. Providing you have done the preparatory work it will be perfectly safe to let your patient take full control at this stage.

Having collected the evidence 'for' and 'against' and successfully eliminated or minimised the evidence 'for', many patients find it helpful to
have the evidence against the delusion written on a card so that they can
use it to counter the delusional idea should it recur in the future.

Example from clinical practice

The example given below is a card developed for a girl who believed she
was evil. Note that the card does not gloss over the 'real' piece of
evidence she produced to support the belief, namely that she would physically attack people when angry, but rather seeks to re-evaluate it. Since it
was more than possible that she would attack someone in the future, it
was important that the modified interpretation of this behaviour was
included on the card.

I KNOW I'M NOT EVIL BECAUSE:

**An EVIL person is someone who *deliberately* wants to make people
suffer and who *enjoys* seeing them suffering. An evil person doesn't do
nice things.**

1. I don't do things deliberately to hurt people. Even when I do
   things when I'm angry I'm sorry later and try to put things
   right. Everyone is unpleasant sometimes during their lives but
   that doesn't make them evil.
2. If I see others suffering I try to comfort them if they want that. I
   don't enjoy seeing people suffering.
3. I get pleasure from seeing other people happy – it makes me feel
   more cheerful when other people are cheerful.

Some of the nice things I've done recently.
1. I swapped a meal with another patient so she wouldn't go
   hungry.
2. I let my room mate listen to her Hindi music before she goes off
   to sleep even though I don't enjoy it.
3. I chatted to a new patient on the ward to make him feel at
   home.
4. I helped Wendy cook some pancakes.

Note that in the above card the term 'evil' is clearly defined, an example
of making a general concept more specific so that it could be challenged
and contradicted by evidence. Beliefs about being evil or the devil are
unfortunately not uncommon, and in these cases we find it useful to

agree with the patient some definition of evil that specifies that the harm or suffering inflicted on others is deliberate and a source of pleasure. For the patient above, specifying that the essential characteristic of evil was that of gaining pleasure from deliberately inflicting harm on others was sufficient to allow her to see that the delusion was not true. However, if the patient had had episodes when she had intended to harm someone else and had got some satisfaction from doing so, then the definition would have been made more extreme, perhaps extending it to include doing harm *all the time* or to *everyone*, and *never* doing anything nice for anyone. In order to get an appropriately worded definition of this or any other delusional belief of this kind, you have to do the exploratory work first to ensure that your patient will not fit the final definition in any way – which is just another example of the therapist doing preparatory work before proceeding formally with the challenge in order to ensure that the challenge, when made, has a successful outcome.

Summary of how to collect and use evidence

1. *Is the delusion based on a strong feeling but little evidence?* If so, the approach is to show that feeling is not the same as fact, that even though this particular feeling is very convincing it could be (and is) misleading.
2. *Is the evidence given in support of the delusion based on someone else's interpretations and beliefs?* If so, the approach is to undermine these dysfunctional interpretations and beliefs and replace them with more functional ones.
3. *Is the evidence given in support of the delusion a distortion of something that really happened or a misunderstanding of someone else's opinion?* If so, the approach is to correct the distorted interpretation or misunderstanding so that it no longer supports the delusion.
4. *Is the evidence given in support of the delusion itself delusional?* If so, the approach is to modify the supporting delusion, using whichever CBT strategies are appropriate, in order to invalidate the evidence.
5. *Collect evidence to contradict the delusion.* Whilst the evidence in support of the delusion is being discredited or minimised, evidence against the delusional belief is collected together with evidence to support the alternative belief; some of this evidence may come from reality testing.
6. *Expose the patient to the contradictory evidence.*
7. (Optional) *Weigh up the evidence for and against.* When the evidence in favour of the delusional belief has been removed or is heavily outweighed by the evidence against it, then your patient can proceed with a formal evaluation of the evidence concerning the delusion.

ALTERNATIVE EXPLANATIONS

Delusional beliefs are developed and maintained as the result of the way the patient interprets his internal experiences and external events. Evidence that is interpreted by the patient as confirmation of his delusional belief can only be undermined if he changes his interpretation, and he will only do this if he comes to see that an alternative interpretation is more likely to be correct. Thus, the establishment of more plausible explanations of events and experiences is a key aspect of the work to modify a delusion. For this to happen, the alternative explanations have first to be generated, and then they have to be shown to be more consistent with the evidence overall and more likely to be correct than the original, delusional explanations.

Following the general CBT principle that it is better if the patient comes up with the ideas than if the therapist suggests them to him, ideally you would encourage your patient to generate the alternative explanations and interpretation of events, taking care in the early stages to treat this as a theoretical exercise only and not making any attempt to push the patient towards accepting any particular alternative or to express your own support for one over another. Ideally, you would then explore the alternatives with your patient, using logical arguments and collecting evidence to test them out. However, in practice, we have found that it is often difficult, if not impossible, to get our patients to stand outside their experiences and to take an objective view of them in this way. Because of the problem we have found in getting patients to generate the alternative explanations and viewpoints, we have developed the practice of floating these past the patient as a way of establishing that alternatives could exist, whilst making it clear that we are not particularly supporting any one of them or indeed doubting the patient's own explanation. Some of the phrases we have found useful in this situation are given below; note that most include a rider that expressly casts doubt about the alternative suggested in order to make it easier for the patient to reject it and to enable you to remain remote and untainted by it.

1. 'I was wondering if ... is that a possibility at all or have I got it quite wrong?'
2. 'Do you think there is any chance that ... or is that not a possibility?'
3. 'It seemed from what you were saying that it could be that ... but have I got that right?'
4. 'Someone else I knew had an experience that sounded a bit like yours and he found in his case that it was due to ... Do you think something like that could be going on with you or is your experience of ... quite different?'

Providing you do not imply support for the alternatives you float past in this way they can be useful sources of information even if they are rejected. Patients will normally explain to you why you have got it wrong and this gives you more information about the evidence that will be needed in order for it to be reinterpreted or re-evaluated.

If for some reason it is not a good idea for you to suggest the alternatives to your patient, for example if your patient is very sensitive to any suggestion that you doubt him, then it may be possible to generate alternatives for discussion by asking your patient what his doctor, nurse, family, etc. think is going on and if they see things differently from the way he does. This strategy does not always work because patients' perceptions of other people's beliefs can be so highly coloured by their own as to be unhelpful, for example 'My mother thinks I need a rest' or 'My doctor's trying to ensure that the hospital stays full so that he gets a fat salary'. However, if your patient is able to report the alternative views of other people you can then explore with him why he thinks they might see things in the way that they do. Note that if your patient is sensitive about your not disbelieving his point of view then you would need to pursue this line gently and slowly, making clear that you are not judging the other people's views one way or the other but are just curious as to why they have come to the conclusions that they have. Occasionally, patients will conclude that the other people can have no good reasons for coming to their (different) conclusions, in which case it is permissible for you to muse that they must have some reasons, reasons that seem valid to them even if they are not valid in fact. You must be careful not to push your patient into believing that if other people have no valid reason then they must be part of a conspiracy against him, but it is important and helpful for your patient to understand that different people can genuinely and honestly see and interpret things quite differently, even though not all the interpretations can be correct in fact.

On rare occasions the patient is so convinced about his delusional belief and explanation for events that he is not willing to explore or even discuss the alternatives suggested. If it is very important for the patient to get a shift in his delusional belief then the only way forward may be for the therapist to inform him of the medical team's alternative explanation and then point out to him why it is necessary to prove whether his or the medical team's explanation is the correct one. The therapist can either adopt the position of puzzlement ('It's really difficult for me to know which view is correct as you both seem to have reasons to back you up') or of reassuring the patient that you are not disbelieving his explanation ('If you are right it would be really important for the doctors to know so that they don't keep you in hospital unnecessarily but equally, if by any chance the doctors could help in any way with what's been going on, then that would be important for you to know'). Having agreed the need to prove which explanation is correct, you are in a position to start collecting evidence and testing things out.

Example from clinical practice

The approach described above had to be used with a patient who believed he was surrounded by evil spirits. This was a terrifying delusion as he believed the spirits could, among other nasty things, cut off his arms and legs. The delusion worried him a lot less when he was under medication because the influence of the spirits was felt less often and was less intrusive but he had a history of being released from Section, being discharged and then immediately stopping medication, only to become very disturbed again and require readmittance and remedication under Section. Some change in the belief about the spirits was considered important, not only to reduce his fear of what the spirits could do to him but also, and perhaps more importantly in this case, as a reason for medication compliance after discharge. He already accepted that the doctors did not believe him about the spirits so we clarified that they believed his experiences were due to some illness. I was then able to discuss with him why I thought it was important for him to get some evidence to try to resolve these conflicting theories: if he was right then it was clearly important for him to be able to prove to the doctors that this was so, so that they could understand and stop giving him inappropriate medication or bringing him into hospital. I also floated the alternative that I supposed it would also be important for him to know if the doctor should, by any remotest chance, be correct because that would imply that it was indeed the medication that helped him when he came into hospital and not just the opportunity to get lots of sleep; but I didn't press the point. Having agreed that it was necessary to find some proof one way or the other, we were then able to move into what evidence, reality tests, etc. could prove or disprove the spirit explanation, an exercise he had considered a sheer waste of time when its aim had been just to prove what he already knew in fact.

Caution: Such a head-on attack should only be attempted as a last resort, after all gentler approaches have failed, and it should only be attempted if it is very important for the patient that he modifies his delusion. As you are effectively forcing your patient to consider the contradictory evidence and alternative belief before he has achieved any insight you must make sure that you have done as much destigmatising work as possible so that the belief change, if it does come about, is not experienced by the patient as just replacing one unpleasant belief with another.

Some alternative interpretations of events will constitute a direct challenge to the delusional beliefs whilst others will not. For example, a patient believed that one of the occupational therapists wanted to prevent him getting better and as evidence for this said that she had not asked him to help her sort out the art materials that morning. The alternative explanations, that she might have wanted the art material laid out differently that morning and so had to do them herself, or that she had not seen him waiting at the door, are neutral alternatives because accepting them as true would discredit this particular piece of supporting evidence but would in no way disprove the core belief about the occupational therapist wanting to prevent his recovery. On the other hand, the alternative explanations, that she did not want him to get paint on his new jacket or that she did not want to tire him out before the painting began, would challenge the core delusional belief because these would imply that the occupational therapist felt positively caring towards him and therefore that she would not want to retard his recovery. You need to be aware of the potential impact of the alternative that you suggest to your patient because you should be more cautious when working with an alternative that actually contradicts the underlying delusional belief.

In general, it is easier to generate and discuss alternative explanations for external events than for internal, subjective experiences. Partly this is because, as we have already noted, subjective experiences, including perceptions and misperceptions coming from our five senses, come imbued with their own sense of certainty. However, another important factor is that we all, understandably, think that we are in the uniquely best position to interpret our own subjective experiences because we are the only ones who are directly aware of them, and therefore we do not take kindly to having our experiences queried by other people. For example, I may disagree with you about whether or not the ball was out during a game of tennis but I will admit that you have as much right to form an opinion about the event as I do; however, I would think you had overstepped the mark if you told me that in your opinion I did not really have the toothache of which I complained. Therefore, if you are suggesting an alternative explanation for a subjective experience reported by your patient you should make it very clear to him that you are not for one moment doubting his experience, but that the alternative you are suggesting is for what caused the experience and not for the experience itself.

Before being able to suggest an alternative explanation(s) to your patient you will have had to generate it for yourself. Whether you offer one or more alternatives depends on what you are hoping to achieve by this exercise. If, for example in the early stages of therapy, you are only wanting your patient to accept that there are possible alternative explanations for most situations, without suggesting that any of these alternatives is more appropriate than the delusional explanation, then you would offer as many alternatives as possible, including some with a low probability of being correct. (You should, of course, be careful not to suggest anything adverse or that would feed into other delusional beliefs.) Giving a number of alternatives not only makes the point more forcibly that other possibilities exist, but also it avoids any suggestion that you are pushing a particular alternative in preference to the delusional one. If, however, you are at the stage of wanting to establish one particular alternative explanation as a more likely alternative than the delusional one, then you should go for just the one that is most likely to actually apply. The 'true' explanation may not seem the most persuasive to your patient, particularly in the early stages, but it will certainly be the most resilient to logical reasoning and testing and to subsequent events in the patient's life, so this is usually the one you would try to establish.

In some cases, it may be difficult for you to ascertain which of a number of possible alternative explanations is the 'true' one, or there may be more than one 'true' explanation (e.g. Patient 1, below). When this occurs, you should float the likely alternatives past your patient, or discuss them with him, to see which he feels are the most likely to be true, and work from there.

Examples from clinical practice

The examples given below suggest some possible alternative explanations for events and experiences given in support of the delusions held by three patients.

Patient 1
Delusion: People know I'm not really human.
Evidence: People were looking at me in a strange way when I went into Epsom (the local town).
Alternative explanations

1. People are looking at you in a normal way but you feel uneasy and self-conscious and so you're oversensitive to them looking at you.
2. It's because you stare at them when you're trying to check out their response to you; they notice you staring at them and are worried why that might be, so they look at you.
3. It's because people in Epsom are not used to people who dress like you – people wouldn't take any notice in London but this is conservative suburbia.
4. It's because you mutter under your breath and that's unusual, so people are worried that you might be very upset about something.

Patient 2
Delusion: There are insects under my skin.
Evidence: I can feel them crawling around.
Alternative explanations

1. It's the tiny nerves just under your skin that are firing off for no parti-
    cular reason, a bit like when you suddenly get an itch, but more so.
    Note: For this patient we could think of only one reasonable alterna-
tive. The possibility of some skin disorder was considered to be an
undesirable alternative and the possibility of irritation from clothing or
bedding was too unlikely and easily disproved.

Patient 3
Delusion: Someone is trying to poison me.
Evidence   The orange squash tasted funny at dinner yesterday.
Alternative explanations

1. The water jug had not been properly washed out.
2. The orange squash was old and had gone a bit stale.
3. The orange squash was stronger/weaker than usual.
4. It was a different brand of orange squash.
5. The warm weather makes things taste slightly different.
6. You had been eating something with a strong flavour that affected
    your taste buds.
7. Your cold/catarrh/hay fever affects the way things taste.

Note: We would have suggested that the medication might be responsible
for changing the way the orange squash tasted if we had thought that this
was the true explanation, but as it was not considered likely it was not
suggested as a theoretical possibility in case it affected the patient's
medication compliance.

REALITY TESTING

Reality tests are situations that are set up for the specific purpose of
producing evidence that is directly relevant to the delusional belief and/or
the alternative belief. Providing they are set up properly, this evidence is
clear and unambiguous and so can be very persuasive.

The aims and detail of a reality test are agreed by the therapist and
patient working together, so it is not possible to engage in targeted reality
testing until the patient has at least some recognition that his delusional
explanation and/or belief just might not be the appropriate one. It would,
of course, be possible to set the patient up to conduct a reality test of a
delusion whilst he is still absolutely convinced it is true, for example by

asking him to do something that would 'prove to other people that his delusional belief was true', but it would be rarely, if ever, acceptable to do so. Not only would such an approach lack honesty on the part of the therapist but also it could force a change in the delusional belief before the patient had been adequately prepared for it.

There are four broad areas in which reality testing can be used.

1. *To test the evidence that supports the delusional belief or on which the delusional belief is based*, e.g. 'I know I have special powers because I can predict the future'. Showing that the patient cannot predict the future removes one of his reasons for believing he has special powers.

The impact that successfully challenging a piece of supporting evidence has on the delusional belief itself depends on how important that piece of evidence is for the delusion. If, as in the case just cited, the evidence is a major reason why the patient believes his delusion to be correct, then disproving it will have a significant impact on the delusional belief and may even be sufficient to bring about a belief change. On the other hand, if the piece of evidence is just one among many then the reality testing may not have any significant effect on the underlying delusion until many such pieces of evidence have been discredited. Where the impact of the reality testing is potentially greater, you must be all the more careful that your patient has been prepared for the disconfirming results and is otherwise ready for the belief modification. Conversely, reality testing of less significant evidence will have less of an impact and therefore can be conducted earlier on in therapy. However, in this latter case you should be careful not to make a big issue of the disconfirming results, because if you force your patient to resolve the inconsistency between his delusional belief and the results of the reality test, he may do so by distorting the interpretation of the reality test results.

Reality testing is essentially concerned with evidence produced in the here and now, but it can also be used to check out interpretations of events in the past. Although the identical situation can never be reproduced, it may be possible to set up a very similar situation so that the results can be used to counter or at least cast doubt on the previous interpretation. For example, it was not possible to disprove that a shopkeeper had made derogatory remarks to one of our patients the previous week, but we were able to reality test his reaction to her on further occasions; as he was polite and pleasant to her on these subsequent occasions we were able to suggest that this made her initial interpretation about her experience less likely and the alternative explanation, namely that it had been one of her voices again, correspondingly more likely.

2. *To directly test the delusional belief*, e.g. 'I can cause you to feel unwell

by ill wishing you'. Showing that the patient cannot affect the way other people feel will disprove his belief in his power to do so.

Where it is possible to directly test a delusional belief, as in the example given, then this is the most powerful reality test to use. Since such a head-on challenge to the delusional belief is capable of bringing about a more or less immediate belief change you must be careful not to conduct the reality test until the alternative belief has been discussed with the patient and is available to take the place of the disproved delusional belief.

Because of the power of a direct challenge to a delusional belief, this is often the final stage of a modification programme, introduced after all the preparatory work has been covered. Logical reasoning and evidence evaluation may cast doubt on the delusional belief whilst a direct reality test can provide the conclusive evidence to clinch the belief modification.

3. *To test an implication of the delusional belief, i.e. a prediction that, if disproved, would necessarily also disprove the belief on which it is based*, e.g. 'If Nurse X wants to kill me then she must hate me: if she hates me she won't help me repair my jacket if I ask her'. Showing that the nurse is willing to help mend the patient's jacket will demonstrate that she does not hate him, and if she does not hate him then it can be argued that she would not want to kill him.

Reality testing of implications is less powerful than directly testing the delusional belief itself because it involves more links in a chain between the delusional belief and the reality test results, and so more stages where the line of argument can be weakened or broken down. For example, in the case just mentioned, if the nurse helps the patient to repair his jacket then this cannot be used as conclusive evidence against the belief that she wants to kill him either (a) if the patient thinks of any other reasons why she might help him repair the jacket other than thinking kindly of him, (e.g. 'She likes sewing' or 'She wants to look good in front of her ward manager') or (b) if he thinks of any other reason why she might want to kill him other than that she hates him (e.g. 'She's being paid to kill me' or 'She's been threatened that something will happen to her family if she doesn't do it').

Some delusional beliefs cannot, by their very nature, be tested directly and so reality testing implications of the belief may be the only option available. Beliefs about the supernatural world usually fall into this latter category, as do delusional beliefs about future events. However, in some cases you may choose to reality test the implications of the belief even if that belief could be tested directly, either because it is a gentler form of challenge than a direct test or because the belief is so strongly held that you want these results to add further weight to the result of the direct test.

4. *To directly test the alternative explanation or belief*, e.g. 'The pain in my stomach is due to indigestion, not the effects of poison'. If the stomach pains after eating can be prevented by slowing down the patient's rate of eating plus the use of indigestion tablets, then this would support the alternative belief that the pains were due to indigestion.

Usually the reality test that is used to disprove the delusional belief will, at the same time, support the desired alternative, but you should not make the assumption that this is so. If the reality test disproves the delusion but leaves open a range of possible alternative beliefs, then before you carry out the reality test you must ensure that the desired alternative is the strongest one available so the belief modification, when it occurs, will be in the direction you have intended.

In some cases it may be more helpful to target the reality test at the alternative belief, rather than the delusional belief, so that the results will actively strengthen the desired alternative belief. If the alternative belief is incompatible with the delusional belief, i.e. only one of them can be correct, then this approach is as effective as a direct test of the delusional belief but may be pleasanter for the patient to conduct, as he will be proving himself right rather than wrong about something. If proving the alternative belief to be possible does not rule out the possibility that the delusional belief could be correct, then testing the alternative belief could be useful as an early strategy but would not be sufficient of itself to eliminate the delusional belief.

Characteristics of a good reality test

It is important that reality tests are set up correctly in order to achieve the desired result. In particular, you must avoid inadvertently providing support for the delusional belief or producing evidence that the patient can interpret as positive support even though most people would not interpret it in this way. Reality tests should have the following characteristics.

1. The result of the test should be clear, precise and unambiguous

It is important that the reality test is set up so that there can be no doubt or debate about what the results were. This means that the outcome must be clearly specified and measurable, and the test must take place within set time limits.

If you do not specify clearly what would count as 'positive' and 'negative' evidence then there is a significant risk that the patient will interpret something else that happens during the period of the reality test in line with his delusional belief and therefore regard this as positive evidence to support his delusion. This is certainly not what you want. Reality tests are set up to test out the delusional belief and to highlight the results obtained, and as such they will tend to magnify the significance of any positive, supporting evidence, should it accidentally occur. We can use the example of the patient who believed he could predict the future to illustrate this point. If the reality test he is set is to predict the outcome of the 2.30 race at Epsom then there can be no doubt about whether or not his prediction was correct. If, however, you have not specified what the prediction of a future event is to relate to, but have left this rather vague, it is highly likely that the patient will interpret some other event as proof of his ability to predict the future, for example, he might have known what type of biscuits were going to be brought into the group meeting that week.

Similarly, if you do not set a strict time limit to the reality test then there is the risk that something will happen weeks later which your patient will interpret as support for his belief, and at a time when you may not be around to discuss the interpretation he has made. For example, if a patient believed that there was a conspiracy to make him ill, then it is likely that he will fall ill with at least a cold or flu at some time in the next year. If the reality test involves something happening within a time limit we usually set the time period to be between one session and the next, though it can be much shorter, i.e. within a single therapy session, depending on what is being tested.

2. The interpretation of the results should be unequivocal

You must ensure that you check with your patient how he will interpret the various possible outcomes of the reality test before putting the test in motion. However convincing a test may be to you, there is no point in running it if the patient would not accept or would be able to explain away the results. For example, one of our patients believed his head was empty, that his brain had been removed. As he was going to have a full neurological examination we suggested the reality test of asking the neurologists for a copy of his head X-ray. We asked how he would interpret the X-ray if it showed a brain in place, like the example from a text book that we were looking at, but he replied that he would not believe it and that if the neurologist said that this was his X-ray then he would know that the neurologists had switched them. So without any prospect of disproving his delusional belief, we did not attempt this reality test.

It is recommended that you and/or your patient make a formal note of the patient's interpretations of the possible outcomes before running the reality test in order to clarify and strengthen them. Having a formal record also helps to prevent the patient discounting these interpretations in favour of some other explanation when the reality test provides the expected contradictory evidence. Even so, should the patient show any unwillingness to accept his pre-test interpretation of the results when they are obtained, be prepared to back off and wait until more work has been done before presenting the evidence again. If you attempt to force your patient to come to a conclusion when there is an apparent reluctance to accept the desired alternative belief then there is a risk that the change he makes will be in the direction of another delusional belief.

Results that are open to different interpretations are not suitable for a reality test and so, wherever possible, the outcome of the reality test should be some publicly observable event or happening about which there can be no differences of opinion. For this reason, subjective experiences can only be used as outcomes if it is possible to make some objective measure of them. For example, it would be possible to set up an experiment to test the patient's belief that he could make other people feel unwell by ill wishing them. The patient would ill wish the therapist for one hour in the week and the therapist would keep a record of how well/ unwell he felt every hour to see if the hour he felt most unwell coincided with the patient's ill wishing him. By recording their experiences, the therapist and patient would convert their subjective feelings of being unwell into an objective and definite event that cannot be reinterpreted later.

Note: In practice the reality test for this particular patient involved the patient and therapist well wishing rather than ill wishing one another: the patient was reluctant to ill wish the therapist because he thought he would be successful and the therapist did not want the patient to think that he would ever wish him ill, even as part of an experiment aimed at helping him in the long run. As a general point, reality tests dealing with pleasant things are preferable to those that could potentially (for the patient at least) have an unpleasant outcome, because they are less stressful for the patient. However, because of the very nature of the unpleasant delusional belief being tested, it is usually the case that one cannot avoid at least some of the possible predicted outcomes being unpleasant ones. Indeed, this is why it is usually necessary to use logical reasoning and evidence evaluation to bring the patient to the point of thinking that his delusional belief is quite possibly, or even probably, not true before he will be willing to reality test it.

3. The probability of a positive outcome due to chance should be very small

Since you are reality testing with a view to disproving the patient's delusional beliefs you must avoid the risk of inadvertently 'proving' that belief with a positive outcome. Therefore, you should specify some outcome that is very unlikely to occur by chance; normally, we reckon that the probability of a positive outcome by chance should be at least less than one in a 100.

Do not assume that your patient will interpret the results as you will, especially when you are dealing with probabilities rather than black and white certainties. For example, if you were conducting a telepathy experiment with four different shapes you might be very satisfied that your patient guessed only 25% correctly, just what would be expected by chance, and consider that this result provided convincing proof that he had no telepathic powers. However, your patient might be able to ignore the items he got wrong but be impressed by how often he did get a correct answer and so take this as proof that he can do telepathy sometimes.

Be careful not to inadvertently risk a positive outcome occurring by chance by over-enthusiastically trying to reinforce the results of a test by repeating it. For example, if you are testing the patient's telepathic powers by asking him to guess a number between 0 and 100, then it is within safe limits to do this once, i.e. the chance of his getting it correct by chance is low enough to risk. But if you were to repeat this a further nine times then the chance of his getting one correct has now gone up to one in ten; too high to risk, as it is unlikely you would be able to explain the statistics of chance convincingly enough to your patient to persuade him that his guessing correctly on one occasion was not significant. Of course, it is perfectly safe to repeatedly test events that could not possible happen, e.g. spontaneous combustion.

If the patient is anxious about the results of a reality test

Although the patient is unlikely to agree to a reality test of his delusional belief unless he recognises that there is at least a possibility that the outcome will be negative, i.e. that it will disprove the delusion, a reality test would not be necessary if he was *sure* the delusion was untrue. Therefore, where the delusion is about some unpleasant or frightening matter, it is to be expected that the patient will approach the reality test with some trepidation. There are two main ways in which you may be able to keep the anxiety to acceptable limits.

1. Although it is usual for the patient to conduct the reality test himself, if the delusion is such that someone else (usually the therapist) could test it out, then this is likely to be much less anxiety provoking for the patient. For example, if your patient believed that alien forces would cause him to spontaneously combust if he said he did not believe they existed, then you could say this loudly and firmly so that he could see what the aliens did to you, before risking the test himself. Although

involving yourself rather than the patient may provide a less conclusive test of the delusional belief, it may be sufficiently reassuring to allow him to then conduct the reality test himself.

2. If your patient is anxious about the possible outcome of a reality test then the test should be carried out and completed during a single therapy session, so that you can support him through his anxiety and remind him of all the logical arguments, etc. that have proved useful in casting doubt on the delusion. Depending on the nature of the delusion, it may be possible to limit the test to a very short period, in the order of only seconds. When the outcome of a short reality test is seen to be negative, i.e. the feared outcome does not occur, then this may provide the patient with the confidence to try longer periods.

Therapist participation in the reality test

If you are taking part in a reality test with your patient you should always carry out your part in the test as agreed, however certain you are that the test will turn out in a certain way. For example, if you agree to well wish your patient for one hour during the week then you should do so, and similarly, if you are supposed to be recording each hour how you feel then you should do this genuinely. This is not just a matter of living up to the trust that your patient has in you to do what you say you will do and of not telling lies to your patient, though these are important considerations. Genuinely testing out a delusional belief is an important part of your acceptance that you could be wrong about it, and your patient could be right.

Example from clinical practice

The delusional belief 'people can read my mind' is a fairly common one in clinical practice. Having someone else read one's private thoughts would be an outrageous invasion of one's personal privacy, so it is not surprising that patients find this belief a very unpleasant one. Added to that, some patients are also worried or ashamed at the idea that other people might know exactly what they have been thinking. If this latter is the case, then it is appropriate to do some normalising work around the content of the average person's thoughts and automatic thoughts, before going on to reality test the accuracy of the delusion itself.

Since this belief is usually based on a strong feeling the patient has that other people are reading his mind, the aim of reality testing is not only to provide convincing evidence that people cannot read his mind but also to provide him with a handy test that he can use on subsequent occasions, to confirm that people are unable to read his mind, should the strong feeling that they can do so occur again.

Before reality testing this particular delusional belief, we usually ask the patient the following questions.

1. *Can you read other people's minds?* The answer to this is nearly always 'no'. (If it were to be 'yes', then you would have to devise a separate reality test to show that he could not, in fact, do this.)
2. *Do you think that I (i.e. the therapist) can read your mind?* Patients usually express uncertainty, but regardless of the answer you can re-assure your patient that you definitely cannot read his mind, though being sure to admit that of course you cannot speak for other people's ability to do so. None of the patients I have reassured in this way has ever doubted what I have said, and apart from any reassurance this statement may give, it also serves the function of being a very gentle challenge to the implication that 'everyone' is capable of reading his mind.
3. *Can other people read one another's minds?* Patients often have to stop to think about this question and usually the answer is 'no'. In this case it may be helpful to wonder how the person's brain could come to be made so differently from everyone else's and, thinking along evolutionary lines, how strange it would be for everyone else's brains to suddenly have developed this power to read just one individual person's brain. Occasionally, the answer is 'yes', the patient thinks that other people can read one another's minds. This can be countered easily by arguing that if people could read one another's minds then they would not need to speak aloud to one another and certainly they would not spend such large amounts on telephone bills!

The reality tests described below are just some that have been used with patients. Some provide more watertight evidence against the ability of people to read the patient's mind than others, but as in all aspects of this work, it is what the patient finds convincing that matters, not what you or anyone else would consider to constitute proof. As you move from level 1 to level 5, the tests become stronger in that the results are less easy to explain away.

If you are going to try any of these tests with a patient of yours, do not forget to discuss with him how he would interpret the different possible results. The general principle is that there is no point in running a reality test if your patient will explain away the disconfirming results obtained, but on the other hand there is no point in conducting a complicated experiment if a simple one will suffice.

Level 1 Ask other people if they can read your mind
This test will be effective only if the patient trusts the other people to tell the truth, but it is perhaps surprising how often patients do accept people's replies to this question, even where there is a paranoid flavour to

their delusions. So in clinical practice, do not forget this very basic reality test; it is very simple and easy to use and can be effective.

The major caution with regard to this test is that the patient should not question people who might give a positive response out of a misplaced sense of humour or for some other reason; in order to reduce this risk you should discuss with your patient who would be a reliable person to question before he does so. Another potential disadvantage of this test is that if it is overused it may become irritating to the people being questioned and this in turn may lead to unsympathetic and even mischievous responses being given. If a reality test is to be used frequently, then it is better if it does not directly involve other people.

Even if a patient initially accepts the results of this reality test, if the strong feeling of mind reading persists then he may come to doubt whether the people he asked were telling him the truth. If this happens he would need to use one of the reality tests given at levels 4 or 5.

Level 2   Conduct a telepathy experiment
This would be set up with the patient attempting to send telepathic messages to you or to someone else who agrees to take part in this experiment. (Of course, if your patient has already accepted your reassurance that you cannot read his mind then you would have to involve someone else as the 'mind reader'.) The test can be set up informally, with the two people together in a session, or more formally, with your patient and the receiver sitting in separate rooms; how you set it up will depend on what your patient feels is the most appropriate and impressive way of conducting the test.

The test stimuli should be something that is very unlikely to be guessed by chance, so four-digit numbers or unusual words are suitable. Do not use common, self-generated words as it is surprising how often words like apple, orange, cat, dog, etc. spring to people's minds, so there is too high a risk of getting a 'hit' by chance. It is also recommended that you do not use drawings for these experiments as it is all too easy to see features of the target drawing in the often rather vague efforts of the receiver.

In fact, telepathy experiments have no more power to disprove that the other person can read the patient's mind than simply asking the other person, because the former, like the latter, relies on the patient trusting that the other person will respond honestly and truthfully. Be that as it may, a few patients do seem to find the formal set-up of a telepathy experiment more persuasive than simply asking the person concerned, so if this is the case then you should conduct the experiment.

Level 3   Think/send a request or instruction to another person and monitor his response
Although the request would be for something that was unlikely to occur without the request being heard, the response itself does not necessarily

have to be an unlikely one, because the most likely response to hearing nothing is to do nothing. For example, your patient could test out a nurse's mind-reading ability by standing at the dinner trolley silently asking for the jam tart pudding option, because even if there are only two options available, the most likely response of the nurse is to ask the patient what he wanted rather than to give him one of the puddings without asking.

The only potential problem with this kind of test is if the patient is in a social situation where he would normally be asking for something, e.g. in a shop, in which case his apparent silence might come across as a bit odd, something that in general you would want to avoid. In order for this not to happen, you should discuss the request and the situation with your patient to ensure that his silence will not be socially remarkable or embarrassing.

As far as interpreting the results of reality tests at this level is concerned, it is quite feasible to explain away the negative results as being due to the other person having read the patient's mind but then he/she not wanting or not being bothered to respond. If the patient argues this way then a higher level test would be needed.

The advantage of this type of test over the telepathy type of test is that it does not require the 'receiver' to know about the experiment in progress or to know anything about the patient's delusional belief.

Level 4   Send a message that is so important that anyone receiving it would respond, and monitor the response

Some patients believe that people will not admit to being able to read their mind because for some reason they want to conceal this fact. The 'reason' for wanting to conceal this fact from the patient can be tackled using the CBT strategies described earlier in this chapter, but especially if the patient is unsure or quite vague about what reasons people might have for such a conspiracy, it may not be necessary to go through this lengthy procedure. If a reality test can provide conclusive proof that people cannot read the patient's mind then the 'reason' why people might be doing it, or concealing that they can do it, becomes irrelevant.

If what the patient is thinking about is sufficiently important to someone else then it can be argued that if the person concerned could read the patient's mind and knew what he was thinking, then they would respond even though it would mean revealing that they had read his mind. Below are some examples of messages of this type that patients have found useful, not only for the initial reality testing of the delusional idea but also as a way of disconfirming the feelings of mind reading when they occur.

1. (To a nurse) 'The hospital/hostel is on fire', 'Patient X is about to abscond', 'You've left your car lights on'.

2. (To someone in the room) 'There's a wasp right behind you'.
3. (To someonoe about to sit up) 'Imagine a drawing pin, spike up'.

If one were being very precise, it could be argued that if other people could really read the patient's mind then they would know that the things he was thinking about were not really happening and so they would not need to respond to the messages they picked up from his mind. In practice, I have never had a patient who argued this way, but if you did, or if there is a risk that your patient might discover this flaw in the inter-pretation of the results some time after conducting the test, then you would need to use a level 5 test.

Level 5   Send a true message that is so important that anyone receiving it would respond, and monitor the response
1. 'I have a £1.00 coin (or £10.00 note), anyone who asks me for it can have it.'
2. 'I have a cigarette (packet of cigarettes), anyone who comes to me and says 'I like Christmas pudding' can have it.'

In order to make these tests watertight the patient must agree to carry out whatever he promises in the message, so in the examples given he would have to have the money or the cigarettes that he was offering to give away.

The big advantage of these tests is that they are simple and easy to do, and as they do not involve the willing participation of anyone else, they can be repeated frequently to counter the feelings of mind reading if this is necessary. The only thing you need to be careful about is that your patient is not sending a message that might be responded to by chance. For example, if he is sitting in a room of cigarette-deprived smokers it would not be advisable for him to send out a simple message 'If anyone asks me for a cigarette they can have it' because it is not unlikely that someone will ask the patient for a cigarette anyway. In this case you would add something very unusual that the 'receiver' has to do or say (e.g. saying 'I like Christmas pudding' in the middle of summer) before they can claim their cigarette.

If perchance the patient had a good reason for thinking that people were concealing their mind-reading abilities despite the advantages they would get from responding to the messages they received (for example, that the doctors and nurses wanted to make out that the patient was ill so that he would have to stay in hospital) it would be easy to argue that such a reason would not apply to strangers, who could only stand to gain by responding to the message, and then conduct the reality test with strangers. (We have never met this line of argument in clinical practice.)

Level 4 reality tests have no advantages over level 5 tests except that they can be used when the patient is not able to carry out the promises of the level 5 tests, for example, if he has no money or cigarettes to give away. In practice, therefore, we now tend to go for one of these level 5 tests straight away in order to disprove that people can read the patient's mind.

CHECKING AND RECAPPING

As with all CBT, it is important to check your patient's understanding of each piece of work that you do, so that you do not press on too quickly or in the wrong direction, or inadvertently present conflicting or confusing ideas and evidence. The art of skilful checking is to do it in such a way that your patient does not feel he is being examined on the work you have covered.

It is standard CBT practice for the therapist to recap frequently, both within sessions and from one session to the next. Not only is this a powerful means of reminding your patient (and yourself) of what you have covered, but it also reinforces it prior to the next therapeutic move. Recapping summarises the work you have covered, allowing you to pull it together within a cohesive framework and giving you the opportunity to emphasise the key points. It is also one way of checking that your understanding of the implications and significance of what you have covered is the same as your patient's, though to be effective, your patient must feel perfectly free to correct what you say.

Because of the fluctuations that can occur with psychosis, with consequent fluctuations in delusional belief conviction and insight, you should be particularly careful when recapping between sessions in case what was agreed last session is rejected or regarded as too challenging for this session. If you suspect that your patient's level of understanding has changed substantially between sessions then it may be safer to ask your patient to remind you of what you had been talking about last session, rather than to risk a recap that may be experienced as a direct challenge.

This may also be a useful strategy if you suspect that your patient has badly misunderstood a line of therapy that you had been trying to pursue. Paradoxically, if your patient's understanding is quite different from your recapping, then he may be more likely to signal agreement, simply because he is too confused or is unable to see how to correct it.

A key feature of CBT practice is to rephrase what your patient tells you and then to ask whether that rephrasing accurately reflects what he was trying to tell you. This is done not only to help you understand your patient's ideas and experiences but also to help your patient to clarify them in his own mind. You should be aware that by rewording and clarifying what your patient is saying and getting his agreement to that rewording, you may be subtly altering his perception or interpretation of events in the direction of that rewording. This being so, you must be careful of the changes you make and go slowly, and always check that you have understood properly. In your eagerness to reach a more rational phrasing, try not to move too rapidly in this direction as this may result in the patient feeling pressured to see things differently, or to his feeling misunderstood. If this does occur, you should be quick to apologise for having got it wrong and make another attempt. Remember that the least challenging reflection is that which uses the patient's own words exactly; but although this is good for rapport, it will not further your understanding of what the patient meant by his words nor help to clarify or modify his thinking about the matter.

DANGER – MODIFYING A DELUSION IN AN UNWANTED DIRECTION

When presented with overwhelming evidence that a delusional belief is not true or possible, there is always a risk that the belief that replaces it will be another delusional belief. This may be a helpful stepping stone towards the ultimate goal for modification, but if the substituted delusion is less amenable to cognitive challenge than the original delusion, or if it has more adverse implications for the patient, then you will have made the situation worse rather than better. For this reason you should always back off immediately if there is any suggestion that the current delusion might be replaced by a more extreme or harder to modify delusion. You should be particularly wary of pushing a patient towards delusional explanations couched in terms of religious or supernatural powers. By their very nature, they are capable of having profound effects on the patient, who is defenceless against them. Furthermore, spirits and aliens may be able to operate in ways that contradict rational argument and scientific experiment and are, therefore, inherently very difficult to challenge with cognitive behavioural techniques!

One of the points that has been emphasised in this chapter is that you should not make a move that could bring about a change in the delusional belief without making every effort to check what that change is likely to be, but however careful you are it is possible to make mistakes, particularly if you are trying to hurry the therapy along. If you do inadvertently push a delusional belief in an unwanted direction you should immediately become more assertive and directive in order to close it down, if necessary retreating to the position of accepting the original delusional belief. Since the patient has only just come up with this new belief or explanation for events it is likely that his conclusions will still be slightly tentative and so this is the time to move in swiftly to counter them. In this situation it is appropriate to disagree with your patient and to state (gently) that you do not think this alternative can be correct and to give all your reasons for thinking so. The following examples are cautionary tales from my own clinical practice.

Examples from clinical practice

Patient 1

This young man was distressed by threatening voices that he believed came from his girlfriend's ex-fiancé, so we undertook a reality test to prove that the voices, which seemed to come from buildings 50 or more yards away, could not be coming from a real person because real voices cannot travel that far. The first set of experiments produced the results I had expected and he seemed quite pleased about that, but the evidence was not enough to change the delusional belief so we agreed to do some more tests next session. I noticed that although he was willing to participate in the second set of tests he seemed less keen than I was expecting, but I failed to appreciate the potential significance of this and carried the test out anyway. When the irrefutable proof was obtained that the voices the patient heard could not be coming from a real human being, and therefore could not represent real threats of harm from the ex-fiancé, I asked him what that implied. He paused before suggesting that perhaps this meant the voices came from the Martians. This was not a helpful modification so I immediately stated that I did not think this could be so (i) because we had tested how far we could hear voices and we certainly would not be able to hear voices from Mars, which is millions of miles away, (ii) because no-one else could hear the voices, which they would be able to do if they were just voices coming generally to earth from Mars, and (iii) because Martians would speak a language of their own, not English.

This case was one of my earliest and demonstrates what can happen if you fail to appreciate that your patient's understanding about his illness may be quite different from your own. The young man concerned had been in hospital for several years and I had been in several assessment meetings with him when his schizo-phrenic illness was discussed and noted that he appeared to be quite unconcerned. So I assumed that he knew he had a mental illness and that this was perfectly acceptable to him: this was my mistake. It was only by discussing the possibility of mental illness as an explanation for the results of the reality test that I realised he was horrified at the thought that his voices might come from within himself because this would mean he was 'mad'. I immediately went into some normalising and destigmatising work around voices and left the results of the reality test until the patient himself referred to them again.

Patient 2

This case illustrates the risk posed by fluctuations in psychosis and consequent fluctuations in insight if these are not detected. The patient and I had been working together for some weeks to identify ways that she might be able to distinguish between her delusional memories, which were very vivid and totally convincing (what we called her 'dream memories'), and real events. For example, on one occasion she was convinced that she and I had been teaching in the same junior school the week before, and on another occasion that we had just come back from a trip to the local shops. One of the ways that we found worked quite well was that when the memory included other people she would ask them if they recalled the events as well, with the agreement that if they did not then this would indicate to the patient that this must be a 'dream memory' rather than something that had really happened.

On the occasion in question, the patient told me that the previous weekend she had been with her mother on a large boat crossing a street in Epsom. In this instance, I could be sure that this was a delusional memory, but rational arguments about the geography of Epsom (which she knew well) were not persuasive for her and so I suggested we phone her mother. Her mother confirmed that she had no recall of such an event and so I asked the patient what this implied. I was dismayed when my patient thought about this conversation and then concluded that the woman she spoke to on the phone must have been a 'double': I had not appreciated that her psychosis had worsened to the point where she was no longer able to question her memories in the way that we had been doing. This was certainly not a desirable shift in belief so I moved to close it down immediately by stating (i) that 'doubles' did not and could not occur in real life, the only 'double' possible was an identical twin but she and all her family knew that her mother was not one of twins, (ii) that the woman who answered the phone had been at her mother's phone number and therefore must be her mother, (iii) that the woman knew who I was, whereas a double would not and (iv) that the woman knew the patient and our plan of treatment, which her mother did but which a double would not have done. We discussed these points until she was convinced that she really had been talking to her real mother and perhaps her mother had just forgotten about the weekend trip. It was safer for her at this stage to have an erroneous memory about being on a boat in Epsom than for her to

open up the possibility that people can have doubles. This latter
would have been a very difficult belief to challenge, and furthermore it could have been damaging to other parts of our therapy, as
belief in doubles could be used to explain so many inconsistencies
that would otherwise be useful in disproving the accuracy of her
delusional memories and of her other, related delusional beliefs.

10

Practical interventions for hallucinations

INTRODUCTION

The techniques described in the next five chapters have been developed for use with auditory hallucinations because these are the most common type of hallucination in our population. Tactile hallucinations are also relatively common in this group; visual hallucinations are less common but do occur in some patients, as do olfactory hallucinations. In principle, many of the techniques used with auditory hallucinations could be adapted for use with these other types of hallucination. The basic approach is the same, namely to accept that the experience of the hallucination is real but then to work with the patient to modify his interpretation of that experience and to limit its adverse effects on him.

Usually you can start to apply CBT to auditory hallucinations more quickly than to delusions because, even if there is a firmly held delusional explanation given for the voices, the phenomenon of the voices can be readily agreed and discussed. Therefore, if your patient is presenting with both delusions and hallucinations, it is usually appropriate to start by tackling the voices. Furthermore, where delusions and hallucinations co-exist it is not uncommon for the delusion to be supported by what the voice is saying, in which case controlling the voices and modifying your patient's interpretation of them will have significant therapeutic effects for the associated delusion as well.

EARPLUG AND WALKMAN®

If your patient is suffering from auditory hallucinations it is usually a good strategy to start CBT by suggesting he tries using an earplug or Walkman® to stop them. This can usually be done as early as your first session because stopping the voices in either of these practical ways does not imply anything about the content or origin of the voices, nor make any challenge to them. The advantage of offering these practical suggestions is that if they work they provide the patient not only with immediate respite from the voices but also, possibly for the first time, the realisation that he has a certain amount of control over them. A secondary advantage is that the practical interventions give you an easy-to-explain reason for seeing your patient over the first few sessions and an opportunity to demonstrate your concern for his distress.

Note: Occasionally, the practical strategies are found to be effective but the voices then command the patient to stop using them. If this happens, it is probably less stressful for your patient to discontinue their use until cognitive work can be done to disempower the voices and their threats (see Chapter 13).

We usually introduce the practical strategies to the patient along the lines that 'Some people find this seems to block voices a bit like yours' or 'You might like to try this out just to see if it helps at all'.

The earplug

A number of patients with auditory hallucinations benefit from putting an earplug in one ear. At best, the earplug stops the voices altogether, though for some patients it works by distorting or reducing the volume of the voices or even by changing the nature of what they say.

We mainly use wax earplugs (Boots 'Mufflers®', cut in half for greater comfort, cost less than £1.50 for a box of ten) because they are cheap to replace if lost or dirty. You should demonstrate how to warm and mould the wax in your fingers before inserting it into an ear, explaining that these are normally used for pop concerts, when using loud machinery, or to help sleep in planes or other noisy situations. Encourage your patient to try the earplug in both the left and right ears, as some do report marked ear preferences. We do not suggest to patients that they try earplugs in both ears at the same time because of the potential interference with everyday functioning, but a few patients have tried this for themselves and found the effects so beneficial that they continue to use them this way. (Sponge-foam earplugs are more expensive but some people find them more comfortable to use, so they should be considered for longer term use where patients find this strategy useful.)

The theoretical explanation for the beneficial effects of an earplug is uncertain. The original theory that inspired their use was that hallucinations might occur when the brain did not accurately synthesise the sounds coming from the two ears, hence blocking the input into one of the ears would prevent this 'muddle' occurring, but this has not been confirmed by clinical observation and research. An alternative explanation is that the distortion in sound produced by wearing an earplug causes the brain to pay particular attention to the sounds coming from external sources and hence diverts attention away from internally produced 'sounds' (i.e. the voices). Since we are only concerned here with the benefits for the patient, the theoretical explanation of why it works is only important in that if the effect of the earplug depends on the brain's response to the novelty of the sound distortion, then this would suggest that the earplug should not be used for long periods, as this may result in habituation to the effect. Over the years we have found in a few cases that this does happen, though only after many months of continual usage. Therefore, we do suggest to patients that they use the earplug only when the voice is bothering them; nevertheless, a few patients are so troubled by their voices that they choose to keep an earplug in all day.

Although earplugs can be very effective in interrupting the voices (indeed, they are effective in most patients who try them), some patients are unwilling to use them, whilst others find them too uncomfortable to use regularly. If your patient is worried about what might happen to the earplug if he puts it into his ear, then it may be helpful to show him a diagram of the ear and discuss its working so that he can see that the earplug cannot get 'lost'. With respect to the discomfort of the earplug, it is recommended that you try wearing an earplug for a couple of hours yourself, as this may help you to understand why patients may refuse to use this method even though it stops the unwanted voices. Apart from anything else, without that understanding it is easy to conclude that the voices 'cannot be that bad' if your patient will not use such a simple method of stopping them.

The personal cassette player (Walkman®)

Almost all patients gain some immediate respite from their voices by using a cassette player with headphones, though when the voices are very troublesome the volume may have to be turned up very loud. As well as being the most effective this is also the most popular way of controlling the voices.

Although there are good theoretical reasons to suppose that listening to taped speech would be more effective than music in combatting the voices, the large majority of patients prefer to listen to music. The type of music does not seem to matter, though there is some evidence that aggressive pop music (e.g. heavy metal) can provoke agitated behaviour and actually increase the voices. Whilst we do not attempt to stop patients listening to music of this type, if this is their choice, we do warn them of the potential risks and help them to carefully monitor the effects on their voices. Very occasionally, patients have reported hearing messages from the words of vocal music, in which case a switch to non-vocal music has been successful.

We have found that the best way of providing cassette players in our unit is to make them available on the wards for people to sign out as and when required. The patients concerned may borrow them at any time, because if the cassette player is only loaned out for the 'voices' then there is a risk that this may lead to false reporting of hallucinations. We provide rechargeable batteries and also have a collection of tapes (which does not include any heavy metal-type music) for patients who do not have their own.

The cassette player probably has its beneficial effect on auditory hallucinations in two complementary ways. First, auditory hallucinations are known to be adversely affected by stress, so if listening to music is pleasurable and relaxing for the patient then this may indirectly result in a reduction in the voices. Second, the cassette player diverts the patient's attention/awareness away from the voices; this is likely to occur at two levels. Patients report that the louder the music, the more effective it is in blocking the voices, suggesting that some of the attention-switching effect occurs at a level that is under neurological rather than conscious control – the music literally 'drowns out' the voices. However, the more meaningful and attention demanding the input, the greater the effect on the voices, suggesting that there is also some attention-switching effect which occurs at a higher level of information processing and control.

Note: Unfortunately, cassette players are not yet available on the NHS as a standard treatment so you may need to seek funding for them from elsewhere. We have been fortunate to receive generous support for our work from our local branch of the WRVS, from our hospital League of Friends and, more recently, from our hospital management. Another potential source of funding, particularly if you are working in the community, is a local charity.

Long-term effects of the earplug and Walkman®

For most patients, the effect of the earplug or Walkman® on the auditory hallucinations is limited to when the strategy is being used and for a short period immediately after use, but for a few patients there appears to be a longer term beneficial effect as well, with a gradual reduction in the occurrence of the voices when the strategies are used over several weeks. In a handful of cases, chronic voices have stopped altogether for many months. These longer term effects are thought to be mediated by a reduction in the patient's anxiety and arousal levels, which is brought about not only by the treatments themselves but also by the sense of control over the hallucinations that these strategies give. Put another way, knowing that you can stop the voices if they become very bothersome reduces your fear of getting them and reducing your fear of getting them reduces their occurrence: a beneficial cycle has been established.

Earplug and Walkman® as the main treatment strategies

Some patients are not bothered by what their voices say, perhaps because the content is insignificant or because the voices are so indistinct that they cannot quite catch what they are saying, yet they find the unwanted interruptions intensely irritating, especially if they continue for long periods unabated. In these cases, where the primary cause of distress is the irritating presence of the voices, then an earplug or Walkman®, if effective, may be all that is required in the way of treatment. For example, one of our patients was plagued by a babble of meaningless words that continued throughout her waking hours. This made her agitated and irritable towards others, causing arguments and even occasional physical assaults. Using an earplug stopped the voices, thereby breaking the negative cycle of voices leading to stress, leading to more voices, leading to more stress, etc.

A few patients want to get rid of their unpleasant voices but keep their pleasant ones. Where the unpleasantness or pleasantness arises from the perceived source of the voice, because of who or what it comes from, it may not be possible to disempower and challenge the unpleasant voices without also disempowering and challenging the pleasant ones. In these cases, a practical way of reducing the voices that does not imply anything about the nature or origin of the voices and which can be targeted at specific voices, e.g. the earplug and Walkman®, may be the only CBT strategy you can use.

Patients who are very difficult to engage in psychological therapy may be unwilling to look at the issues around the content of the voices so in these cases, even where you believe that CBT could benefit them, these practical strategies may be the only treatment that they want to become involved in. For example, one of our patients was bothered by a voice of unknown origin which would comment on and criticise his actions. Although what the voices said suggested that he was concerned about his standard of performance of everyday tasks, the earplug was so effective in blocking them that he did not want to pursue any further therapy.

OTHER PRACTICAL WAYS OF REDUCING THE VOICES

As part of your assessment, you should ask your patient if he has found or noticed anything that affects the voices, anything that seems to make them better or worse. Many patients will have already discovered something that seems to help, in which case you may be able to work with your patient to ensure that his coping strategy is used more regularly and more effectively. Since these are strategies that he has devised himself, it is safe to work with them from the earliest stages of therapy.

At an appropriate stage of therapy, you might suggest to your patient that he could try one or more of the practical strategies described below as a possible way of helping to reduce his voices. The correct time to introduce these strategies will depend on the patient's beliefs about his voices and the extent to which these practical strategies may 'challenge' these beliefs. For example, learning to switch the voices on and off is likely to constitute an effective challenge to any delusional belief that the voice is independent of the patient, and as such should not be attempted before the patient is ready to accept the belief modification entailed, namely that his voice is not from an external source but is coming from within himself. Where there is full insight about the voices (e.g. 'They're part of my illness' or 'They're coming from me') then all these practical strategies can be used with impunity.

If the voices are so persistent that they occur for much of a therapy session then your patient will be able to try out some of these strategies whilst he is with you, but often they have to be tried between sessions with your patient reporting back on how effective he found them to be. If you are able to set this up as a formal experiment, with your patient noting down the time and place when he heard the voices, what he did in practice and what were the effects on the voices, then this will help not only to determine the effectiveness of the method used but also to demonstrate this effectiveness to the patient. A more severely ill patient is unlikely to be able to follow such a formal task, but nevertheless he will almost always be able to report back whether or not the strategy 'helped' with his voices.

It is usually best to try just one of the practical coping strategies at a time so that you can determine which are the more effective for your patient and then build on them. As you go through the different strategies that patients have reported to be helpful, you will notice that some appear to be exact opposites; for example, concentrating and distracting attention from the voices, or increasing and decreasing levels of stimulation. People are very individual in the way their voices respond to the different coping strategies, which is why it is necessary to try them to see what effect they have for your particular patient.

Subvocal speech or singing under one's breath

Talking out loud is an effective way of blocking auditory hallucinations but it may not be socially acceptable for the patient to suddenly start talking to himself, for example if he is walking along a shopping street or sitting alone on a railway station. In order to avoid social embarrassment, the patient may be able to use subvocal speech, i.e. talking quietly to himself so that no-one else can hear. The theory is that providing that there are minor movements in the vocal chords this will be sufficient to prevent the vocal chord movements that accompany at least some auditory hallucinations. Some patients do report beneficial effects for subvocal speech but one of the major practical obstacles is that patients find it difficult to understand the concept of subvocal talking and are unable to put it into action. Singing under one's breath is easier to under-stand and to do, and as such may be preferable to subvocal speech, even though there are theoretical reasons for supposing that it would be less effective. Another major practical difficulty is that keeping up a flow of subvocal speech requires concentration and effort, so it is only suitable for use over short periods. Repeating sequences of numbers (e.g. 1–10) may be less attention demanding but quickly becomes tedious; subvocal singing may be less effective but it is easier to keep up over longer periods.

Despite the limitations of subvocal speech and singing, this may be a useful practical strategy if it is important to stop the voices and there are no other means to hand, for example if the patient is in a public place when the voices start and he has no earplugs or Walkman with him.

Concentrating/focusing on the voices

In some of the early clinical work with hallucinations, patients were asked to complete homework assignments recording details about their voices when they occurred. It was found that in some cases focusing on the voices in this way seemed actually to reduce the frequency of their occur-rence, so this exercise is now used therapeutically.

The reduction in voices may occur, in part at least, because adopting a scientific/objective attitude to his voices helps the patient to distance himself from them and the power that they have over him, so you should make the exercise as 'scientific' as possible for your patient. The normal way of doing this is to use a formal chart for recording details about the voices when they occur, which you go through with your patient in the next therapy session. A secondary gain from this exercise is that the additional information about the voices that it provides may suggest other coping strategies; for example, the patient whose voices occurred most frequently in the television room decided to avoid this room until his voices got better.

Focusing does not work for all patients and not all can complete this type of formal homework assignment, but as it can be beneficial it is worth a try, providing your patient does not become more agitated or distressed in the process. This may occur if the content of the voices is very unpleasant, especially if one of the patient's coping strategies is

avoidance. In these cases you should work on the content of the hallucinations (see Chapters 12 and 13) before asking your patient to concentrate on his voices outside the safety of the therapy situation. You can
test out the distress level caused by concentrating on the content of the
voices by asking your patient to do this within a therapy session, though
you should remember that the distress caused is likely to be quite a bit
higher when he is on his own, without your support, and when the voices
are actually speaking the content aloud.

Switching the voices on and off

Some patients are able to bring on their voices within the therapy session.
It may not have occurred to them to try this before, so asking them to
imagine the voices talking may help to bring them on. Once the voice has
been voluntarily produced in this way the patient tries to turn it off
again, either by fading it away or by terminating it suddenly. Having
practised switching off the voices that have been produced voluntarily,
some patients are able to transfer this learnt ability to switch off the
voices when they occur involuntarily. This technique is not suitable for
patients who do not have insight into the origin of their voices, and so
should not be used either before insight has been achieved or in cases
where full insight is not the desired goal of therapy. Although in our
clinical practice we have had little success using this technique, because
the few patients for whom it was appropriate have been unable to
produce their voices voluntarily, there are reliable reports in the research
literature that this technique can work, so it is worth a try; it may be that
the technique is more appropriate for less severely ill patients.

Although voluntarily producing the voice has irrefutable implications
about its origin, the same is not true for dismissing a voice that has
occurred involuntarily, and so this latter can be used whilst there are still
delusional ideas about the voice. Some patients do report that they can
sometimes get rid of their voices by telling them to go away, though the
relief is generally short-lived. Commanding the voice to stop seems to be
more effective if shouted out loud, but because of the social difficulties
this may cause it is worth practising to see if your patient can gradually
reduce the volume until he can stop the voice by just saying the
command word quietly to himself. This may be particularly important as
some patients find that swearing at the voices in a disrespectful way (e.g.
'f ... off') is more effective than telling them politely to stop.

Restricting the time spent listening to the voices

A variant of the above is that some patients are able to limit the intru-
siveness of their voices in their everyday lives by setting aside a set period

in each day when they will listen/respond to them. Having set aside this time, they are able to ignore or refuse to listen to the voices at other times.

Distraction – games, socialising, TV, etc.

The most commonly reported strategies discovered by patients to help control their voices involve some sort of distraction. Any activity that engages the patient's attention and concentration is potentially suitable for this purpose, but there is some evidence to suggest that activities involving the use of language are particularly effective. This is probably because the speech/language areas of the brain are involved in auditory hallucinations and so using these areas for some other language activity prevents them being used to produce hallucinations. For the same reason, activities that require the patient to talk are potentially better for blocking hallucinations than activities in which the patient only listens. The more attention required from the patient, the more effective the activity will be as a distraction, but this has to be balanced with the problem of engaging the patient in a demanding task, which can be a particular problem for patients with negative symptoms of schizophrenia.

The patient should be encouraged to try various activities, e.g. going to talk to someone, reading a book, playing Scrabble, watching TV, etc. when the voices are troubling him and then to report back any effects these may have had.

Physical activities – brisk walk, run, etc.

Some patients report that engaging in some physical activity helps to reduce their voices; in these cases the physical activity seems to have some beneficial effect over and beyond that of mere distraction, though it is not clear how this effect may operate. Therefore, as with the other activities, you may suggest to your patient that he tries a physical activity when he hears the voices to see if it helps at all.

Reduction in stimulation/stress – relaxation, bed, be alone, etc.

Hallucinations are more likely to occur when the patient is aroused. Although we tend to think of stress and arousal in a negative way, in this context even pleasurable arousal, such as a family gathering or antici-pated pleasure of an outing, can lead to an exacerbation of the voices. If the hallucinations are linked with arousal levels, then some form of relaxation training may be appropriate.

Even in non-psychotic people 'voices' are more likely to be heard in noisy surroundings, and some patients find the best way of coping with their voices is to withdraw to a quiet place on their own. For patients in hospital or busy hostels the only place where they can relax away from noise and stimulation is likely to be their beds, so in these cases retiring to bed in the daytime should be recognised as a legitimate coping strategy and not as a sign of lethargy or negative symptoms that needs 'treating' with stimulating activities.

11

The promotion of insight about hallucinations

INTRODUCTION

The general approach to the promotion of insight about hallucinations is essentially the same as that used for delusions, so this present chapter should be read as a sequel to Chapter 7.

Auditory hallucinations can be upsetting in different ways and for different reasons, so it is important to assess why your patient's voices are disturbing him so that you can plan the most appropriate line of treatment. We noted in the previous chapter that voices can be unpleasant because of their sheer irritant value, but for most patients their voices are particularly distressing because of what they say and/or because of who is thought to be saying it. Although it is often possible to work on what the voices are saying in a way that does not challenge the delusional beliefs about where or who they come from, the general guideline is to carry out some general preparatory destigmatisation of schizophrenia before working on the voices themselves, if there is any risk that this latter work will trigger an unwanted insight or the wanted insight too early. The most usual end goal for insight promotion is for the person to understand that the voice comes from within himself and to understand why it says the things that it does. However, if the goal of choice is to leave intact the delusional belief about the voice's origin then, needless to say, no attempt would be made to promote insight about the voice coming from the patient or resulting from an illness.

DESTIGMATISING AND NORMALISING THE HEARING OF VOICES

As with delusions, insight about the patient's hallucinations is developed within a normalising framework, which in this case means regarding the hearing of voices in schizophrenia as an extreme form of what is an essentially normal phenomenon, a phenomenon which is of no importance in itself and that only matters if it bothers or upsets the hearer. Some of the exercises you can do with your patient to help to normalise and destigmatise the hearing of voices include the following.

Sharing experiences of voices

As with the sharing of 'odd ideas' (see pp. 84–5), sharing with your patient any experiences of hearing voices that you may have had will help to demonstrate that the actual hearing of voices as such is not weird and nothing to be ashamed or frightened of. Whether you are doing this work as part of a group discussion or during an individual session, it may be helpful to know of some other people's experiences to back up your own, particularly if your own are not very impressive. The examples of hearing voices given below are those reported by people on our CBT courses who have agreed that they may be shared with patients.

1. A mother, in an empty house, heard 'Mummy' being called.
2. Someone walking in the country on a windy day twice heard his name being called from behind.
3. A student working one evening heard 'Go out and enjoy yourself'.
4. The same student about to leave his room heard 'Go back and finish your work'.
5. A therapist often heard her own thoughts spoken aloud.
6. A woman heard her recently deceased husband talking to her.

Although most non-psychotic people hear only isolated words, some people do hear phrases and sentences and even continuous speech, much as people with schizophrenia can do, though they have no other signs or symptoms of a psychotic illness. This phenomenon can be disturbing when it first occurs but most 'hearers', as they are sometimes called, learn to recognise and accept their voices for what they are. Studies to investigate the prevalence of voices in non-psychotic people have come up with different results, but some suggest the incidence could be above 70%. In one study, around 15% of the people reported that they often heard their thoughts being spoken out loud. In a recent meeting of psychologists a show of hands indicated that between 70% and 80% had heard voices at some time in their lives. Whether psychologists are particularly prone to voices or whether they are just more willing to admit to it I do not know, but these figures clearly show that hearing voices is really quite common and as such quite normal. It can be very helpful to share these figures with your patient; certainly most patients find it both surprising and reassuring that the incidence of voices in the general public is so high.

When sharing your own experiences of voices you should make clear that you are not suggesting that your voices are the same as your patient's voices, or that they are as disturbing or as distressing. If your patient believes that his voices come from some external source then your aim at this stage is just to demonstrate that it is **possible** for the brain to mishear things. If he is not ready for full insight you should be careful to avoid implying that his hallucinations are the same sort of voices as those that you are talking about.

Discussing the factors that increase vulnerability to voices

The factors that increase the likelihood of non-psychotic people having delusion-like ideas also increase the likelihood of hearing voices (see p. 85). Your patient may be interested to know that most people, if deprived of sleep for only 48 hours, will begin to hallucinate, demonstrating that it is really quite easy to push the brain into this state. Voices are also more likely to occur in noisy surroundings, especially where there is a loud and monotonous background noise with no foreground noise clearly discernible above it, e.g. sitting under a hair dryer, mowing a lawn or in a party. Your patient may have found that his hallucinatory voices are more frequent in some situations than others and be able to recognise some of these factors as being relevant for him.

Education about automatic thoughts and the psychological processes involved in belief formation and maintenance

As we noted in Chapter 7 (pp. 86–90), education about automatic thoughts is essential when working to modify delusional beliefs about the origins of the hallucinations if your patient would be shocked, disgusted or ashamed on discovering that the voices came from within himself. The key points for your patient to understand about his voices are:

1. the voices are not under his control and so 'he' cannot be responsible for them;
2. voices do not necessarily reflect what the person is 'really like'; the voices can utilise anything we have ever learnt about, fact or fiction;
3. voices that produce a strong emotional response are more likely to recur in the future: frightening, shaming or unpleasant voices may be recurring for this reason, not because they are the product of some basic personality characteristic or because they are true.

When discussing voices that recur in the same words or themes, it may be helpful to discuss the phenomenon of obsessional thoughts with your patient. At the time of writing, the similarities and differences between obsessional thoughts and recurrent hallucinations are a matter of unresolved debate but whatever the outcome, the fact that in the obsessional disorders thoughts that do not reflect the person's wants and wishes can recur, outside the person's control, demonstrates that the non-psychotic brain is also capable of functioning in this way.

Discussing the meaning of schizophrenia

See Chapter 7, pp. 92–4.

EXPERIENCE IS NOT THE SAME AS FACT

This aspect of the insight work is very similar to that used for delusions, the aim for hallucinations being that your patient comes to understand that even though his voices sound very real and as if they are coming from outside him, this does not mean that they are coming from some external source, i.e. to understand that his brain is capable of misleading him in this respect.

Misinterpretation of everyday events

When working with hallucinations it is particularly helpful to highlight the everyday misinterpretations that can take place around perceptions; these may include misperceptions of sight and touch as well as of hearing (see the first seven examples on pp. 94–5).

Misperception at a physiological level

Since hallucinations are themselves misinterpretations that occur at some physiological level, this aspect of the insight work is particularly pertinent for voices. The following misperceptions have proved useful with our patients.

Visual illusions

In our version of this exercise we show the patient a number of visual illusions, each one printed on a coloured card (see Fig. 11.1 for examples). In each case we ask him what he sees and then invite him to discover his 'mistake' by using a shape or measure cut from a piece of differently coloured card. For example, in the first illusion shown in Figure 11.1 a piece of card the same shape and size as the two (identical) shapes on the illusion card is provided for the patient to lay over the shapes in the illusion: this clearly demonstrates that the shapes are, in

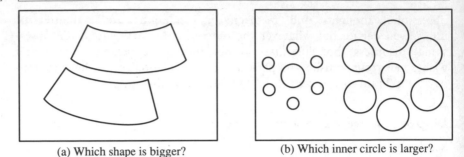

(a) Which shape is bigger?   (b) Which inner circle is larger?

Fig. 11.1   Examples of visual illusions used to show that the brain can mislead.

fact, the same size, even though the top one looks bigger than the lower one. When your patient responds to the illusion, it is important that you agree that the figure looks bigger to you, too. You should do this before you give him the piece of card to check his response so that when he finds he is mistaken then it is clear that you have been mistaken too. Your aim is not to make him feel foolish for making an error but rather to be curious about why this occurs.

Having noted how interesting it is that our brains can misinterpret what they see in this way, we usually offer some sort of explanation for each of the illusions used, in order to make the point that there are perfectly good reasons why, on occasions, the brain can misinterpret what it sees and hears. The explanations we give for the two illusions illustrated are as follows.

In illusion (a), the lining up of the left-hand edges of the two figures suggests that the double figure is actually stretching backwards into the picture: this perspective suggests that the top figure is further away than the lower one. The two figures are actually the same size, so the images they make in the eye are the same size. But the image that an object makes in our eye gets smaller the further away the object gets, so if two objects at different distances make the same-sized image in the eye, then the object that is further away must be bigger.

In illusion (b), when the centre circle is surrounded by smaller circles the contrast in size makes the centre circle seem bigger, whilst when it is surrounded by larger circles the contrast in size makes the centre circle seem smaller.

Note: Readers wanting to construct their own set of visual illusions will find examples and explanations for the illusory effects in most introductory psychology text books.

Pressing one's eyeball

Pressing one's eyeball from the side will produce immediate distortions in the way objects are perceived. (This effect is stronger if the other eye is shut.) As the eyeball is pressed, objects can be seen to 'move'. This effect occurs because pushing the eyeball distorts the lens in front of the eye so that the image of the object on the back of the eye moves, misleading the brain into thinking that the object itself must have moved.

Stick in water

If an object, such as a stick, is half immersed in a glass of water it looks as if it bends at the surface of the water. This is because the light waves are bent as they leave the water, so it looks as if the bit of stick under the water is also bent. (The light waves bend as they leave the water because water and air have a different density.)

Tinnitus

If your patient knows of tinnitus you can use this as another example of how the brain can hear something, in this case a constant whistling, buzzing or rushing noise, which is not actually there. In cases of tinnitus the nerve that normally conducts messages about sounds from the outside world becomes damaged and so it sends off messages all the time, misleading the brain into thinking that they are real sounds coming from the outside world.

Phantom limb

This is a very useful example for showing how the brain can misinterpret where something is coming from because of the way in which the brain assumes that if a particular nerve is active, this must mean that a particular area of the body has been stimulated. For example, a patient who has had a lower leg amputated might feel pain in his right toe even though the foot no longer existed. This is because the nerve that would have ended up in the right toe has been activated at the point where it was cut off at the knee. As far as the brain knows, this nerve still ends in the right toe and therefore it 'feels' the pain as located in the right toe.

Some patients feel that they ought to be able to control their voices if they come from within themselves, so these examples of persisting misperceptions from everyday life are particularly useful to demonstrate to them that the higher, rational parts of the brain are not able to override the misperceptions of the more automatic parts, and therefore that it is not possible for them to override their 'hearing' of the voice.

Use of dream analogy

Whilst we are dreaming, we are not aware of anything abnormal about what we are hearing in those dreams. We are convinced it is real sound, even though we realise on waking that it was not.

DISCUSSION OF HOW AND WHY THE VOICES MIGHT HAVE OCCURRED

The perceptual experience of the voices

We use slightly different explanations for the perceptual experience of hallucinations, choosing whichever seems to fit in best with the patient's own conceptualisation and is the most appropriate. The way in which you present these explanations and the detail that you go into should be adapted so that they make sense to your patient.

Auditory hallucinations as mis-attributed inner speech

When we think, we can sometimes be aware of using words and talking to ourselves in our thoughts; this is sometimes called 'inner speech'. Scientists have now shown that parts of our brain that we use when we talk and listen to other people are also used when we are producing this inner speech. Since some of the same areas of the brain are involved when hearing our own thoughts as when hearing other people talking, it may be relatively easy for the brain to make the mistake of attributing the words used when thinking to some external source. Once the words have been erroneously attributed to an external source, then the subjective experience would be to 'hear' them as real sound (cf. the phantom limb, p. 183). The diagram given in Figure 11.2 is a simple representation of this explanation and this, or some adaptation of it, may be helpful in showing the patient how easy it would be for the brain to make such a mistake.

Auditory hallucinations as vivid automatic thoughts

If you do not want to enter into a discussion about inner speech with your patient, you can explain the occurrence of auditory hallucinations more simply in terms of automatic thoughts that are so vivid and strong that the brain misperceives them as having come from outside. The term 'automatic thoughts' is used in preference to 'thoughts' to account for the patient being unaware of having generated them.

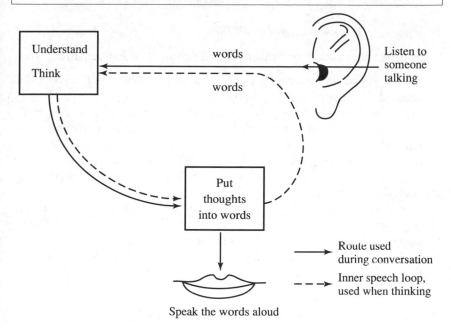

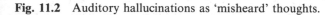

Fig. 11.2 Auditory hallucinations as 'misheard' thoughts.

Auditory hallucinations as the result of interhemispheric interference

It has been suggested that some auditory hallucinations may occur because the information coming via the left and right ears is not co-ordinated correctly in the language area of the left hemisphere and this 'muddle' results in inaccurate (i.e. hallucinatory) perception of external noises. Whilst this theory has not been entirely confirmed by clinical and research evidence it may be a helpful explanation for those patients whose voices tend to occur in noisy surroundings.

The form taken by the voices

In order for your patient to get greater insight into his hallucinations, he needs to know not only how they could be produced at a physiological level but also why they have taken the form that they have, i.e. why they say particular things and why they appear to come from a particular person or entity. Your explanation about the form that your patient's hallucination has taken will be very specific to him.

Why does the voice say what it does?

Some of the more common reasons for the content of hallucinations are:

1. that it reflects an underlying worry, fear or concern (e.g. the voice that accused the patient of being overweight);
2. that it is something the patient read about, heard or saw that frightened him or seemed important to him for some other reason (e.g. the voice that threatened the patient with spontaneous combustion);
3. that it reflects the patient's belief about something; this belief might or might not be delusional (e.g. the voice that said Dr X was trying to poison the patient);
4. that it is a memory of something that has happened to the patient (e.g. the voice that accused the patient of being a 'pervert and queer', using the same terms and tone as someone from his past);
5. that it is just a vague idea that floated through the patient's mind (e.g. the voice that told the patient he was a 'superimposed crackerjack').

Why does the voice sound like somebody known to the patient?

The usual explanation given for this is that the part of the brain that has learnt to recognise different people's voices is wrongly activated during the hallucination so that the brain thinks it recognises the voice as the person concerned. Since this involves tapping the memory for what different voices sound like, voices that are more familiar or are of more importance for the patient are particularly likely to be inappropriately activated and hence 'recognised'. Similarly, voices that have been heard recently by the patient will be fresh in his memory and therefore more easily activated.

Explanations in terms of memory, be they memories of real past events or of heard about or imagined events, seem to be particularly useful for some patients in making sense of their voices. We sometimes refer to them as 'fragments of (distorted) (inaccurate) memory, that have got stuck on a broken record and so keep coming round and round'.

Example from clinical practice

It may be important for your patient to have a good, solid explanation for his hallucinations so that when the voice recurs he can use it to counter the more obvious explanation, namely that the voice sounds real because it is real, and also so that he can counter what it is saying. For example, one of our patients explained his recurrent voice along the lines 'I was very upset when Joan accused me of being fat and ugly so it made a big impression on me; also, I'm worried that I've got a bit overweight so I'm particularly sensitive on the issue. Therefore, if my brain 'mishears' the thoughts flashing through my mind, it is particularly likely to latch on to anything to do with food and weight, and this is likely to trigger my memory of what Joan called me so vividly that I hear her voice saying the same things as she said to me then'.

12

CBT with the non-psychotic beliefs influencing the content of the hallucinations

INTRODUCTION

Hallucinations are not randomly produced words and sentences, they are produced by the patient's brain and so it is not surprising if they reflect his concerns and beliefs about himself and the world. These concerns and beliefs may be accurate with respect to the objective world, for example the overweight patient whose voice accused her of being a fat lump, or inaccurate, for example the patient whose voice accused him of being evil and the patient who was accused of having had a hundred babies. It is important that you assess how accurate your patient's voice is or could be, because this will affect the emphasis you put on the different aspects of treatment and, crucially, the order in which these aspects are tackled.

IF WHAT THE VOICE SAYS IS UNTRUE

If what the voice is saying is clearly **not** true in fact, then you can proceed to directly challenge it, confident that by so doing you will be able to disprove what it is saying (see Chapter 13). Of course, this does not mean that you should neglect to tackle any dysfunctional beliefs that may underlie what the voice is saying, only that it does not matter what order you do it in.

Example from clinical practice

One of our patients was accused by her voice of being mentally retarded. Since this was clearly not true, we were able to set about disproving the accusation straight away, which was easily achieved with a combination of logical reasoning and evidence collection (see p. 195). This had some effect on the frequency of the voice but it still occurred from time to time. We felt it was likely that the voice reflected some underlying fear that she might be retarded, even though she was unable to come up with any reason or evidence to base this on. So whilst she was using arguments and evidence to successfully counter the voice whenever it said she was mentally retarded, we were constantly alert in our sessions to pick up any comment or hint as to what might underlie the fear, because whilst that fear was still present we predicted that the voice would continue to recur from time to time.

After several weeks we picked up the missing links: she believed that 'too much sex makes you demented' and also believed that she had been promiscuous in the past. Having elicited these two underlying beliefs we were able to modify them using the standard CBT techniques of logical reasoning and evidence gathering. We discussed the old-fashioned belief about over-indulgence in sex and dementia, and agreed that it came from the times when syphilis was the cause of the dementia. She did not believe that she had syphilis. We also used the arguments that married people, who have sex regularly, do not die earlier with dementia than single people or nuns, and that there were not large numbers of ex-prostitutes in the elderly dementia wards of our hospital (fortunately she did not require proof of this; she knew some of the patients and knew that they had been in hospital for very many years, so their opportunities for sex would have been very limited and certainly less than the national average).

The patient herself was not promiscuous and had not been promiscuous in the past, but this was her underlying fear. We explored this issue and she was able to readjust her evaluation of herself. As it turned out, her sexual activity was probably below the average for her age, so she was able to use this in another line of reasoning to counter the fear, which went 'Even if it were true that too much sex makes you demented (which I know it's not because of all the reasons and evidence we found that proved it wasn't true) I have not had more sexual contacts than other women of my age, so even in days gone by that old saying would not have applied to me'. (Of course, if there had been a history of frequent promiscuous sexual contacts then we could not have 'disproved' this particular belief about herself, in which case we would have had to rely on the arguments and evidence to show that sex and early dementia/ subnormality were not related in order to break the dysfunctional chain of thinking.)

This case is a good example of how work with hallucinations and delusions may set off a chain of CBT work that encompasses areas unrelated to the psychosis as such. In this case, the content of the voice suggested that the patient might be concerned about her sexual behaviour, now or in the past, so this led to CBT work with her underlying beliefs about sex and sexual relationships.

IF WHAT THE VOICE SAYS IS TRUE

If what the voices are saying is true, then it will not be possible to disprove them; in such cases the most effective line of treatment is likely to be modification of the beliefs surrounding what the voices are saying. For example, in the case of the patient whose voice accused him of being fat it was not possible to challenge the voice on the accuracy of what it was saying, because he was significantly overweight, so the only way to reduce the distress caused by the voice was to attempt to modify his beliefs about fatness being a matter for scorn and derision. We did not discuss dieting with him for fear that this would imply that we agreed with his voice that fatness was undesirable and shameful and that it would be better if he were thinner. From his past history, we could be fairly certain that dieting would not work, so it was certainly not worth risking inadvertently supporting his dysfunctional beliefs about fatness when there was only a very low chance that he would be able to reduce his weight by dieting.

When the content of the hallucination is true, it is important that you tackle the underlying beliefs before you try to disempower the voice or modify any delusional ideas about its origin, because tackling the voice directly may imply that you agree with the underlying belief. (**Note**: You can offer an earplug or Walkman® as a temporary way of stopping the voice whilst you are working on the underlying beliefs, because their effectiveness implies nothing about the voice or its content.) In our experience, once the patient is no longer bothered by what the voice is saying, because the underlying belief has been modified, then the voice stops saying this particular thing, or only says it very rarely indeed. For example, in the case mentioned above, if the patient no longer worried about his weight then he would no longer be distressed by the voice's comments, and so one of the maintaining cycles would have been broken.

Unfortunately, though perhaps to be expected, the beneficial effect of targeting a specific underlying belief does not seem to generalise to other things that the voice says, so the voice continues to say these other things. If these are also supported by underlying dysfunctional beliefs then these have to be similarly targeted for modification.

Example from clinical practice

One of our patients was distressed by persistent voices calling her 'whore' and 'prostitute'. This had been occurring for many years and it had become the practice to reassure her that what the voice was saying was not true. The beneficial effects of this reassurance were short-lived and she would seek reassurance again, wearing down the patience of the staff in the process. The problem was that, unknown to the staff caring for her, there had been a time in the past when she had attempted prostitution, only on a couple of occasions but nevertheless often enough to provide some support for what the voices were saying. This being so, simple reassurance was not appropriate and could not be successful in the long term. Furthermore, implicit in the reassurance given by the staff was confirmation that they believed reassurance was appropriate, i.e. that it would be insulting to be accused of prostitution because being a prostitute would, indeed, be shameful.

Since the voice's accusations were related to a true incident and reflected her feelings of shame at what had happened, it was decided to tackle her belief that 'Prostitution is wrong and so anyone engaging in an act of prostitution should feel guilty'. First, we looked at what was meant by the term 'wrong' and came up with the definition that morally wrong meant doing something deliberately to hurt or offend against someone else. We then looked to see who had been hurt by her actions and concluded that she was the only one who had suffered in any way, by her feelings of guilt and regret. Hence we concluded that her acts of prostitution had not been morally wrong and therefore that she should not feel guilty for them.

We were aware that if we successfully modified the patient's belief about prostitution being morally wrong this would remove what might be an important factor in controlling her present sexual behaviour, so at the same time as we looked at the moral issues around prostitution we also looked at the practical side. We went through the health risks associated with prostitution (we also took the opportunity of doing some safe-sex education) and considered other disadvantages of the lifestyle, for example the risk of being a victim of violence and the fact that some people, whether rightly or wrongly, do disapprove of prostitution and prostitutes. We also included in the list of disadvantages the fact that her past history indicated that she would be very worried afterwards, for weeks if not months, that people would find out about it.

Having looked at the advantages and disadvantages of prostitution for her, she decided that the disadvantages were much too high a price to pay for the few packets of cigarettes that prostitution would bring her. We noted that most women come to similar conclusions, though for a few people the advantages seem to outweigh the disadvantages and so they chose to become prostitutes. The final conclusion from this exercise was 'Prostitution is not morally wrong; if that's what other women want to do that's OK, but it wouldn't suit me because I would worry so much about the risks that it just wouldn't be worth the money I'd get'.

She still blamed herself for what she had done when she was younger and all the subsequent upset it had caused her, so we also looked at the context of her brief move into prostitution so that she could better understand why it had happened. We considered why it had seemed like a reasonable option at that time, understanding and knowing what she did then, and why she felt differently now. This enabled her to view her young self less critically and with more sympathetic understanding.

Viewing the acts of prostitution in the past as potentially unwise (though fortunately no physical harm had come to her), rather than morally wrong or shameful, took the sting out of the voices' accusations and this may have been an important factor in their reduction. We also involved the care staff in the treatment so that instead of reassuring her on the rare occasions when the voice did recur with this particular accusation, they would adopt a more neutral attitude of 'I don't know whether what the voices are saying is true or not, but it wouldn't matter to me one way or the other'.

IF YOU ARE NOT SURE WHETHER THE VOICE IS TRUE OR NOT

Because of the importance of not directly challenging the content of a hallucination if it is true, if you are in doubt it is safer to treat the content as if it were true and to attempt modification of surrounding beliefs before tackling the hallucination *per se*. For example, one of our patients was accused by a voice of being a 'gay queer'. He vehemently denied that he was homosexual, but in view of his strong negative beliefs abut the subject it would have been very difficult for him to acknowledge any inclinations that way. So even though there was no evidence to suggest that he was homosexual, we considered it safer to attempt to modify his underlying beliefs about homosexuality being disgusting rather than seeking to show that what the voice said about him was untrue. If he were exclusively heterosexual then gathering supportive evidence would have been a quick and easy way of countering the voice and reducing the distress it was able to cause, but there was a significant risk that taking this approach would imply our tacit acceptance or even approval of his negative views of homosexuality. Furthermore, if it had turned out that the patient did, indeed, have homosexual tendencies, then this would have compromised our position to carry out what would in these circumstances have been the most effective element of the treatment, namely to modify his beliefs about homosexuality.

IF THE PATIENT IS WORRIED ABOUT THE IMPLICATIONS OF HEARING VOICES

Some patients may not be concerned by what the voices say so much as the implication of hearing the voices. For example, one of our patients was primarily concerned about her voice because she knew that 'hearing voices' could be a sign of schizophrenia. She was horrified by this notion because she believed that if she had schizophrenia this would mean that she might suddenly go berserk and kill someone. In this case blocking the voice with an earplug or Walkman® might have provided some temporary relief from stress by allowing her to avoid the voice, and this might even have led to a reduction in its occurrence, but her fears about madness and running amok would still have been there to be triggered whenever a voice occurred. The more effective treatment for the distress caused by her voice in this case was to modify her underlying dysfunctional beliefs about schizophrenia and hallucinations. Not only did this reduce the anxiety and fear caused by the voice when it occurred but also, because she no longer had to avoid the thought that she might be mentally ill, this enabled her to consider the issue of medication more rationally.

| 13 | **Disempowering the voices** |

INTRODUCTION

Although auditory hallucinations are subjective in that they come from within the patient's own brain, they are experienced by him as being objective phenomena and so he is able to stand apart from his voices in a way that he is not able to do with his delusional beliefs. This means that, in most cases, it is easier to talk to your patient about his voices than about his delusions. Furthermore, you can form an alliance with him against the voices and challenge their power and authority head on, whereas challenges to delusional beliefs usually have to be much more subtle and oblique. Therefore, if your patient's voice is saying something unpleasant it may be possible to move quickly to challenge and discredit the content, with the major provisos that (i) if the voice is accurate in what it says it will probably be more appropriate to work first with the patient's non-psychotic beliefs underlying the content (see Chapter 12) and (ii) if a successful challenge to the content would have implications for the patient's delusional explanation about the source of the voice, then this should not be done until after the preliminary insight work has been covered and the patient is prepared for the belief change should it occur. For example, if a patient believes that God speaks to him and tells him about the future, then proving that the voice cannot predict the future as claimed could have a significant impact on his belief that the voice was from God; hence you would not challenge the voice in this way until the patient was ready to shift his belief about the voice coming from God.

The main aim of working directly with the content of hallucinations is to discredit and disempower the voice, so that even if it says nasty things the patient is not frightened or otherwise unduly upset by it. Although the voice may still be an unwanted irritant it will have no greater impact on the patient than that, and reducing the distress caused by the voice usually has the secondary effect of reducing the frequency and duration of the voice. One or more of the following strategies, as appropriate, may be useful in disempowering the voices.

EVIDENCE TO DISPROVE WHAT THE VOICES SAY

If what the voices are saying is not true then it should be possible to prove that they are wrong by the use of logical reasoning and contradictory evidence. However, as a first step you need to find out if the patient has any reasons or evidence that the voice could be telling the truth, so that these can be discredited. Especially where the voices relate to delusional beliefs, it is quite possible that the patient has misinterpreted events in such a way that they support what the voice is saying.

The content of the voice can be subjected to logical reasoning and evidence collection in the same way that delusions are (see Chapter 9). The contradictory evidence can be built up from anything the patient has noticed in the past that seemed to be inconsistent with what the voices said plus evidence collected during the course of therapy and from reality testing. When you have collected all the evidence and arguments against what the voice is saying, the most persuasive pieces can be summarised on a card for your patient to carry with him, to help him challenge the voice when it 'speaks' outside the therapy session.

Remember that even where the content of the voice is clearly untrue, it may well reflect some underlying concern or dysfunctional belief. Therefore, you should try to ascertain what the underlying beliefs might be and then treat them as appropriate (see Chapter 12).

Example from clinical practice

The card reproduced below was made for the patient described in Chapter 12 (pp. 188–90), whose voices accused her of being mentally retarded. The evidence included was couched in her own words and represented the items she found most convincing. Item 3 on this list was not produced

---

I am not mentally retarded because:

1. I can read and write.
2. I can have a normal conversation with another person.
3. I've got an 'O' level in French and sat for 8 other 'O' levels (therefore I must have been brighter than those pupils who didn't sit for exams – and this was a normal school for *non-retarded* children).
4. I have good personal hygiene - I can look after myself.
5. I can cook, shop, etc.
6. If the nurses tell me I'm not retarded, then I'm not. They have been working with me so that I can get a true understanding of my condition and have not told me lies about anything else.

---

spontaneously by her, but as it was possible that at some time in the future she would encounter people with learning disability who could read and write, have a normal conversation, good personal hygiene, etc. the more solid evidence about her academic achievements at school were elicited from her for inclusion. (**Note**: With respect to Item 6, we do encourage patients to rely on their own reasoning abilities rather than asking other people for their opinions, but in this case the patient wanted to include this as a piece of hard evidence and so it was included.)

THE VOICES CANNOT HARM

Threatening voices are particularly disturbing and frightening, so the primary aim here is to disempower them, to show the patient that they cannot cause him any physical harm. The treatment approach is essentially the same as for any other delusional belief.

Making the general specific

In order to plan the most appropriate strategies, you should try to find out from your patient exactly what the threats are. In general, specific threats are easier to disprove than vague, nebulous ones.

In some cases your patient may be so frightened of the voice, or so frightened of what will happen to him if he talks about it, that he is unwilling to give you any details. If this is so, then it is better to work as best you can with the notion of 'something awful' being threatened than to risk raising your patient's anxiety levels even higher by persistent questioning. Once the therapy has started to be effective then it is likely that your patient will feel safe enough to risk telling you more.

In some cases your patient may be unsure of what the harm could be but has a general feeling of the voice's power and its malevolent intent. The general approach in a case like this is the same as if more specific harm has been specified, though the nebulous nature of the harm may make it harder to pin down and disprove. Since it is easier to show that the voice cannot harm your patient physically than mentally or, even worse, spiritually, in trying to make the general specific with respect to the harm being threatened you should avoid pushing your patient towards the notion of mental or spiritual harm. Wherever appropriate, you should accept and agree that the harm threatened is physical.

Discrediting any supportive evidence

In our experience, the power of the voices nearly always lies in the fear of what they might do and not in what they have actually done in the past. However, you must ask your patient if he attributes any ill fortune or unpleasant incident in his life to the action of the voices, because if he does then you should seek to discredit this evidence as soon as possible. Presumably the voices did not really cause the ill fortune so it should be possible to modify his misinterpretation by using logical reasoning and looking for alternative explanations for the events/experiences concerned. In some cases it may be possible to check out some of these alternative explanations even though the event happened in the past, for example, by asking other people who were present for their recollections and interpretations of the events. It is important to disprove or at least cast significant doubt on any evidence that seems to support the voices' power, not only as part of the overall strategy to modify the patient's belief in the voices' power but also to reassure him about the likely safety of conducting a reality test of the voices, later on in therapy.

If, in the past, your patient's voice has set a particular time limit for delivering the harm, e.g. 'I'm going to get you before next weekend' but nothing has happened, these incidents are potentially very useful for therapy. At the very least they prove that the voice tells lies (see next section) but also they can be used to argue for the alternative belief, namely that the voice is not able to carry out its threats.

Logical reasoning

One line of logical reasoning that can be used to show that the voices cannot cause harm concerns the impossibility of non-physical voices interacting with physical objects or bodies. First of all, you need to agree with your patient that his voice is not a solid physical object. I have never yet had a patient who believed his voice to be solid but should there be any doubt you can easily confirm that the voice is not made of atoms and molecules, in the way that objects and people are, by pointing out to your patient that he has never seen the voice or been able to touch it and that it can get to him through solid walls and doors even when he is in an enclosed room. You can then discuss with him how physical objects, including all parts of his body, are made of atoms and molecules that are tightly bound together so that only another object, also made of atoms and molecules, could force its way in between and separate them, e.g. a knife cutting through an apple. Since the voice is not made of solid atoms and molecules there is no way it could cut or otherwise physically affect a solid object like the patient's physical body.

Another supporting line of logical reasoning is to draw a clear distinction between what the voice says and what it can actually do. This distinction may seem rather obvious but in fact even many non-psychotic people exhibit this sort of magical thinking, for example when they feel slightly uneasy about putting their fears into words in case this should make it more likely to happen, so it is worth demonstrating to your patient that saying is not the same as doing. One way of doing this is for you and your patient to say things and then note that what you say does not happen, because you have no power to make it happen, for example 'I am going to turn your hair green in the next five minutes', 'I am going to make you float up to the ceiling' and 'I am going to blow that tree down'. It can be argued that, similarly, just because the voice says it can harm the patient does not mean that it has the power to do so. (More scientifically minded patients may find it helpful if you are able to explain why you are both unable to do what you said, for example explaining the biochemical changes that would have to take place for hair to reflect green light and the power that would be necessary to uproot a tree.)

The evidence and logical reasoning work can often be summarised along the following lines: 'The voice has never managed to carry out any of its threats in the past, so that strongly suggests that it is just not able to do so; it's easy to say something that is quite impossible to carry out'.

Reality testing

As with other delusional beliefs, reality testing the voice can provide impressive evidence of its inability to cause harm. Unfortunately, because of the patient's beliefs about his voice it is highly unlikely that he would be willing to put it to the test, but fortunately he has an ally who holds a different set of beliefs, namely the therapist. So, one of the most powerful techniques for disempowering a voice is for you to issue a direct challenge to the voice to harm you in the way it is threatening to harm your patient – for example, challenging the voice that is threatening to cut off your patient's arms and legs to cut off yours instead. If the harm threatened by the voice is vague then you must specify what constitutes 'harm', making sure that it is something that is very unlikely to happen by chance (I usually use 'Before I see you next week, an accident that is so severe that I will be in hospital for six months') and then lay down the challenge to the voice. If the voice threatens death I do not usually challenge the voice to kill me as this can be rather stressful for the patient; instead, I challenge it to do me some serious harm, like the accident example, on the grounds that if it were powerful enough to kill me it would certainly be able to cause me serious harm.

Normally, you would summarise why you do not think the voice can do as it threatens, before issuing the challenge. You must make it clear that you are taking full responsibility for the challenge and for any harm that comes to you as a result. Even so, the patient may be so fearful of the voice's power that he will become very anxious on your behalf, waiting for the harm to befall you. In these circumstances you should try to limit the anxiety by setting a short timespan for the harm to befall you, for example within this therapy session or the next five minutes, and by limiting the extent of the harm to be done, for example, challenging the voice to cut off your little finger rather than a whole arm. When the feared harm does not happen to you this provides convincing evidence that the voice is not all-powerful; indeed, you can argue that the results are more consistent with a voice that has no power at all, except to frighten the patient by making idle and empty threats that it cannot carry out.

Some patients concede that the voice cannot affect the therapist but are still concerned that perhaps it could affect them. In this case, you can argue (i) that the power of the voice must be very limited indeed if it could only affect one human being, (ii) that the patient's body is made up of exactly the same stuff as the therapist's and therefore it is difficult to see how it could affect the patient's body but not the therapist's and (iii) the fact that it has never actually harmed the patient in the past now looks as if this is because it was not able to do so. If your patient suggests that perhaps the voice did not want to harm you, then it may be helpful to repeat the challenge in such a provocative way that no self-respecting voice would be able to ignore it, for example: 'I think the voice is just an empty bag of wind, making threats it can't carry out', then to the voice 'Come on, if you can cut off my arm do it in the next five minutes – but you can't, can you? All you can do is make empty threats'.

The big advantage of reality testing the voice on yourself, apart from the obvious one of causing much less distress to your patient, is that you can do it very early on in therapy, even when the patient himself firmly believes it to be telling the truth. Proving that the voice cannot inflict the harm that it threatens has two additional spin-offs. First, it provides evidence that what the voice says is not always true and therefore, by implication, that the voice is a liar (see next section). Second, it demonstrates that you are a strong and safe partner for your patient in his battle against this voice.

Example from clinical practice

It is often helpful to prepare a card for your patient summarising the arguments and evidence found useful in countering the voice's threats so that he can refer to it should the voice threaten again. An example of such a card is given below.

When the voice threatens to harm me, I know it can't really harm me because:
1. Only something physical, like a knife or a bullet, can harm my physical body. But the voice is not physical, so it can't do me any physical harm; all it can do is scare me.
2. It's often threatened to harm me in the past, but it never has.
3. When my therapist challenged the voice to harm her badly enough to put her in hospital it wasn't able to do that, so it can't really harm anyone.

Note: When you start challenging voices to harm you in this way you may experience some slight apprehension, especially if the voices are believed by the patient to come from the Devil or some other evil force that is compatible with your religious or cultural beliefs. This feeling of unease should disappear as you collect evidence from your own practice to confirm that other people's voices cannot harm you in any way; this is another good reason for clearly describing exactly what you are challenging the voice to do to you, namely to avoid the risk that you will misinterpret bad luck in a superstitious way. Needless to say, if you would feel too uncomfortable or too vulnerable challenging a particular voice, then of course you should not do so, though you might wish to examine your own underlying beliefs, using CBT principles, to discover why you feel this way about something you are so sure is a symptom of an illness!

The 'owner' of the voice cannot harm

In a few cases, the owner of the threatening voice can be identified as a real person, known to the patient, and it is this person who is thought to be capable of delivering the harm and not the voice as such. For example, one of our patients heard her ex-husband threatening her and she believed that it was her ex-husband who would carry out this threat, not his voice. In such cases the most effective way of disempowering the voice is to modify the delusional belief about its origins, i.e. so the patient no longer believes it comes from the person concerned (see Chapter 14).

Modifying the delusional belief about the voice's origin may take some time or may not be achievable, so it may be worth attempting to reduce the distress caused by the threatening voices by using one or more of the following lines of argument:

1. that the owner of the voice is unaware of what the voice is saying;
2. that the owner would not be able to carry out the threat in practice;
3. that the owner would not attempt to carry out the threat because the penalties he would have to pay would far outweigh his gains.

THE VOICES ARE LIARS

Showing that your patient's voice tells lies, even if it is only for some of the time or on some occasions, can be an effective way of reducing its authority and importance. If the voice tells lies, then your patient need not believe it when it threatens or says unpleasant things about him. The fact that it tells lies can be used at either a reasoning level, e.g. 'The voice has said things that were not true in the past so it may well be untrue now, too' or as a direct confrontation to the voice, e.g. 'You've told me lies in the past so why should I believe you now?' (see next section).

Your patient may be able to recall incidents in the past where his voice said something that turned out later to be untrue, in which case this can be used as evidence that the voice tells lies, but often patients seem unable to recall incidents of this sort. This being so, it is often more fruitful to collect evidence for the voice being untrue or inaccurate from incidents that occur during the course of therapy. Your role in this exercise is to detect and challenge the accuracy of the voice when it appears to be 'lying' and then to gradually collect this evidence together.

Example from clinical practice

The example given below is of a card built up during the course of treatment to show that the patient's voices lied about many things. Underneath each incident of lying is one of the key pieces of evidence that was used to show that they lied.

The voices are liars – in the past they have said:
1. That N.R. is Hitler.
   (Hitler would be over 90 years old if he were alive today.)
2. The nurses wanted to keep me on the locked ward so they would get extra pay.
   (Nurses' pay is fixed however many patients they have.)
3. I am mentally retarded.
   (I can read, cook, look after myself, etc.)
4. I was the only person alive in the universe and that everyone else was a ghost.
   (I can *see* everyone else around me, alive.)

It is good to get as many examples of the voice telling lies as possible, and in some cases it may be possible to provoke the voice to tell lies or make a mistake by questioning it directly (see next section, on questioning the voices). On some occasions the voice may tell the truth, but fortunately it is not necessary for the voice to always or even usually tell lies to be able to use this approach to counter the voice. Providing the voice has lied on at least one occasion, an element of doubt can be introduced along the lines 'The voice has lied to me in the past and so could be doing so again now'.

Inaccurate voices can be labelled as 'liars' or 'ignorant' depending on which view is more helpful for your patient. Where the voice is critical of the patient or accusing him of something, it may be more helpful to attribute the lies to ignorance, because if the voice is ignorant then its opinion of the patient is not valid and not worth having. Whether or not the voices are called liars or ignorant, they can be described as unreliable, not to be trusted and not worth attending to. (See also the section on how to gently mock the voices, p. 205).

DIRECTLY QUESTIONING AND CHALLENGING THE VOICES

In some cases it is appropriate, and indeed can be very effective, for the patient to talk to his voices and question them directly. Talking to the voices may help the patient to distance himself from them, to see himself as separate from them, and daring to directly question and challenge the voices may give him a greater sense of command and dominance over them.

Since the voices come from within the patient's own brain, in order to prepare for what might happen when they are questioned and for the responses they might give, you should always ask your patient the same questions first, so that you can deal with any relevant issues that may arise. For example, a patient who is ashamed of having read pornography magazines in his youth might be accused by his voice of being a pervert. If you are not aware that this is the patient's underlying concern and you encourage him to argue with his voice, then you may be exposing him to the risk of being taunted by the voice with this 'evidence' of his perverted behaviour. Your priority in this case would be to modify the underlying beliefs about reading pornography, so that if your patient did want to challenge the voices directly, later, then he would be able to do so from the security of his new beliefs.

Questioning the voices can be useful in two different though related ways. First, it can be a way of gathering more information about the possible beliefs or memories that may underlie the content of the hallucinations, when the patient is unable to access it or is reluctant to report it. If you are still seeking information about the voice's content this probably means that you are still not sure what it is based on, and whether there is any element of truth to what is being said, so initially the questions should not be delivered in a confrontational way. Furthermore, your patient should only question the voice in this way whilst he is with you, so that any unexpected material produced by the voice can be dealt with therapeutically.

The second reason for directly questioning the voice is that if it is unable to give a satisfactory reply to the questions then this may significantly undermine its authority and power. The more certain you are that the voice is inaccurate in what it is saying and that your patient has no evidence, distorted or otherwise, to support it, the more certain you can be that the voice will not be able to answer the questions put to it and therefore the more assertive and challenging your patient's questioning can be.

Two types of questions are commonly used to interrogate the voices. The first challenges the voice to provide supporting evidence for what it is saying and the second aims to 'trick' the voice into revealing that it is not who or what it claims to be.

'What evidence have you got?'

Where the patient has been unable to come up with any evidence to support the voice's claims or any reason why it might be saying what it is, the voice may be asked to provide this evidence, for example 'What evidence have you got...?' or, if a more confrontational style is appropriate, 'Prove it'. This is a no-lose approach for the patient because there are potential therapeutic gains whether or not the voice 'answers' the questions.

Since you would not have embarked on direct questioning of the voices for the purpose of information gathering until you had established that your patient was not able to provide this information, it is not surprising that by far the most common response of a voice subjected to this type of direct questioning is silence. The inability of the voice to answer the patient back is very empowering for the patient, who has effectively taken control, and not surprisingly it often renders the voice 'speechless' for beneficially long periods (e.g. more than an hour for a voice that previously had criticised virtually non-stop). Once it has been established within the therapy sessions that the voice is not able to answer your patient's questions then he can use this as a strategy to counter the voice outside the sessions, as a way of silencing the voice for a while and/or as a way of demonstrating that the voice is spouting empty words that it cannot back up.

If the voice should answer the patient's questions then the answers given can be dealt with in the CBT programme just as any evidence produced by the patient would be. For example, one of our patients was troubled by a voice accusing him of being evil but we could find no reason for him to believe this and so he asked the voice directly if it had any evidence to prove it. His voice replied that he was evil because he smoked too much. Perhaps it is not surprising that we had not elicited this explanation by normal interview procedures, because we would not have been alert to the possibility that smoking could be viewed in this light. Interestingly, the belief seemed to have developed as the result of an antismoking campaign and confusion about the meaning of the word 'bad'. The patient had taken on board the message 'smoking is bad' and his subsequent line of reasoning seems to have gone: 'Smoking is bad, therefore if I smoke I am bad; bad means evil, so if I smoke I am evil'. Having uncovered this confusion we were able to draw a clear distinction between 'bad' meaning physically harmful and 'bad' meaning morally evil, as a result of which the voices became less frequent and then disappeared altogether.

'Do you know...?'

The second type of question is used by the patient to expose that the voice is ignorant or does not always tell the truth. Since your aim in asking these questions is for the voice not to answer correctly, you must be careful that the questions could not be answered from your patient's own knowledge store or by chance or guesswork. The principle is to ask questions whose answers the voice ought to know but that your patient does not, for example asking the voice of the Archangel Gabriel how many Christians there are in China. As a precaution to ensure that your patient does not know the answer you should ask him the question before he puts it to his voice, and as a precaution against lucky guesswork on the part of the voice you should ask your patient to have a guess at what the voice might say in response to the question.

In order to construct a suitable question you may need to do some research to discover some indisputable fact that your patient can quiz his voice about. The most common response is for the voice to say nothing, which you should interpret as evidence that the voice is unable or unwilling ('unable' is usually stronger) to accept the patient's challenge, both of which put the patient in a superior position to the voice. Similarly, if the voice should give a wrong answer then this can be interpreted either as deliberate lying or as evidence that the voice is ignorant.

If the voice is silenced or makes errors in answering questions it ought to be able to answer, then this may also be used to challenge the delusional belief about the origin of the voice (see Chapter 14, pp. 216–17). For example, the patient who believed his voice came from President Bush asked the 'President' for his wife's maiden name: when the voice was unable to answer, this was interpreted as suggesting that the voice was not President Bush after all.

GENTLY MOCKING THE VOICES

If, through any of the approaches described above, the voices can be shown to be weak, ineffectual, ignorant, wrong, liars, etc. then this will help to overcome the patient's feelings of awe and powerlessness in their presence and give him a sense of control or even superiority over them. It may be helpful to encourage your patient to express his lack of respect for his voices in words, for example 'The voice just tells lies', 'It doesn't seem to know what's true and what's not true', 'It just burbles away making idle threats' or 'It can't answer any of the questions I ask it'. It may be appropriate to enhance the patient's sense of superiority to the voices by noting how much better than the voice he is at thinking and arguing about the issues concerned, for example 'When I argue with the voice it never wins' or 'It can't think about the issues or argue about them as well as I can'.

Whilst encouraging your patient to feel superior to the voices you must be careful that neither you nor he mock them in any way that could be interpreted subsequently as mocking the patient, if and when he reaches the understanding that these voices come from within himself and not from some external source. One way of retaining the patient's sense of superiority over the voices and the confidence and self-esteem that this may bring, whilst not demeaning the patient for being the source of the voices, is to describe the voice in terms of a lower level of brain functioning, rather like automatic thoughts and dreams, and contrasting them with the high-level, rational thinking of the patient himself.

VOICES CANNOT COMPEL ACTION

Voices that give instructions can be particularly damaging for the patient, and/or other people, if he is unable to resist carrying them out. Instructional voices, like other voices, seem to come with their own imbued sense of significance and power, so they may be difficult or impossible to resist even though the patient does not want to behave or act in that way. The patient's ability to resist the voice can be enhanced by disempowering the voice and by altering the balance of advantages and disadvantages of complying. If your patient is trying to resist the voice's instructions then this suggests that there are at least some good reasons from his point of view for refusing to obey. Equally, if he does sometimes comply, then this suggests that there are some advantages or benefits for him in obeying, even if these advantages are not immediately apparent. In this respect, responding to the instructions given by the voice is no different from any other piece of behaviour, i.e. the person will only act if the advantages of acting outweigh the disadvantages, albeit the balance may be tipped in favour of the 'advantages' for only a very brief time.

In order to change the balance of advantages:disadvantages for obeying or disobeying the voice you need to know what these are, from your patient's point of view, so this is very important information to get from him. Therefore, your questions should include not only what the voice is instructing him to do but also whether he tries to resist it and if so how difficult this is, how often he succeeds in resisting it and whether he has developed any strategies of his own to help him to do this. Two other very important questions are what happens when he does obey the instructions (or, if he has never obeyed, what he thinks would happen if he did) and also what he believes or fears will happen if he resists and does not obey. When collecting this information, do not forget to include the very important effects that obeying and resisting the instructions may have on the patient's emotions, as well as the more obvious, objective results of his behaviour. Having obtained this information you would seek to remove as many of the advantages of obeying as possible, while attempting to build up the advantages of resisting.

Removing the advantages of obeying the voice

A patient may find it difficult to detect or report the advantages of obeying the voice, especially if he normally tries hard to fight it and if the resulting behaviour is disapproved of by himself and others, so it is important to be non-judgemental and accepting about these advantages. Indeed, it is often appropriate to explain to the patient why his behaviour is perfectly understandable in the circumstances even if it is undesirable for social or other reasons.

If there is a delusional fear that the voice can somehow harm your patient if he does not obey, then your first step is to remove this very powerful reason for obeying it, following the approach discussed in the section 'The voices cannot harm' above. A simple but powerful argument in this context is 'The voice would not need to tell *you* to do that (e.g. cut your wrists) if it was able to do that for itself'.

Some voices may have to be obeyed because of who or what they come from; for example, if the voice is seen to come from some powerful spiritual or alien force then your patient may consider it right and proper for him to obey its commands even if they conflict with his conscience or normal behaviour. In these cases it is usually necessary to modify the patient's belief about the origin of the voice in order to remove its authority over him (see Chapter 14).

For many patients, one of the major advantages of obeying the voice is that it stops bothering them, at least for the time being. This being so, if the voice can be stopped in some other way, e.g. by using an earplug or

Walkman, then this can effectively remove one of the reasons for obeying it.

In some cases, it may be possible to remove the advantages of obeying the voice by other means. For example, a patient who followed her voices' instructions to hit her fellow patients when they pestered her for cigarettes identified two advantages of this behaviour: the patients concerned stopped putting her under pressure and she gave fewer cigarettes away. Assertiveness training produced the same end results and so effectively removed these particular reasons for obeying the voice.

Increasing the advantages of resisting the voice

Theoretically, increasing the disadvantages for the patient of obeying his voices' instructions should also reduce the probability of his responding, but for ethical reasons it is not considered to be appropriate to involve punishment in a treatment programme. Nevertheless, there are usually naturally occurring 'punishments' that result from obeying the voice, so you should make sure that your patient is well aware of these. For example, a patient who hits another patient will have to face questions about his behaviour from staff, may have his medication increased, may have his hostel place cancelled, may have to be transferred to a more secure ward, may have feelings of regret, may disappoint his family, etc.

In some cases it may be feasible to positively increase the advantages of resisting the voice's instructions by using a behavioural programme wherein not following the voice's instructions for set periods would be rewarded in some way, perhaps by interest and social praise from staff or by something more tangible like money or an outing. If an alternative behaviour can be found which helps to provide some of the advantages associated with obeying the voice, then it will help your patient to resist his voices if you positively reward this alternative behaviour. For example, if the patient finds that talking to staff is an alternative way of reducing the feelings of tension associated with the voice then the patient should be positively rewarded for seeking out a member of staff, for example by ensuring that the member of staff will always take time out from what he is doing to sit down with the patient.

It is helpful to consider the advantages and disadvantages of obeying and disobeying the voice in terms of short- and long-term effects, since it is common for there to be short-term gains for obeying the voice, often around reductions in feelings of tension or compulsion to act, but long-term disadvantages resulting from the behaviour itself. In this case, one of the ways of attempting to control the patient's behaviour is to help him to become much more aware of the long-term effects and to bring these consciously to mind to counter the short-term gains when he is tempted to obey.

Your patient may find it helpful to write down the advantages and disadvantages of obeying his voice so that he can refer to this when the voice is actually instructing him.

Weighing up the advantages and disadvantages of obeying the voice

As with all cost/benefit analysis work (i.e. weighing up the advantages and disadvantages of something) it is important that you are unbiased with respect to the outcome and do not start off with the assumption that it is 'a bad thing' for the patient to obey his voices, even if the resulting behaviour appears to other people to be undesirable. For example, one of our patients felt so much better after obeying his voice's instruction to smash a hole through the wooden fence surrounding the hospital that it seemed unreasonable to try to prevent him doing this unless we were able to find another way of reducing his feelings of severe tension when they occurred.

When compiling the list of advantages and disadvantages, it is generally better to concentrate on the advantages and disadvantages as they affect your patient rather than as they affect other people. For example, if the undesired behaviour is hitting another person then it is better to concentrate more on what effect that will have for your patient, e.g. losing the person's friendship, being hit back, being taken back into hospital, etc. rather than concentrating on how much it might hurt the other person. This approach makes it clear that in doing this exercise you are primarily concerned for your patient's well-being; furthermore, it is a fact of life that people are particularly concerned with how things affect themselves and our patients are no different in that.

Questioning the voice: 'Why should I do that?'

The strategy of talking directly to the voice (see pp. 202–4) may also be used to disempower voices that instruct the patient to do things against their will. The question 'Why should I do that?' will either render the voice mute, in which case it can be argued that the voice must be empty and mindless (unlike the patient, who is able to exercise his superior reasoning powers about these issues) and therefore not to be taken seriously, or the voice will give a reply, in which case the 'reason' that it gives can be dealt with as part of the CBT programme. When the patient feels more confident with respect to the voice and its power he may find it helpful to challenge it more assertively, for example 'Why should I put my hand through the window? It's easy for you to tell me to do it because it's me that will feel the pain, not you' or 'If you want someone to punch the nurse on the nose you do it – but you can't, can you? You need me to do it for you, you've got no power'.

Example from clinical practice

The example given below shows the advantages and disadvantages of obeying a voice that 'advised' the patient to punch out windows and cut his arms on the glass.

	Advantages	*Disadvantages*
Immediate	Voice goes away Feel good, less stressed (lasts about 5 minutes) Attention from nursing staff	Pain Staff cross with me
Long term	Feel people are more interested in me as a patient	Arm hurts for several days I can't go out for walks or to the shops Wife gets upset with me Feel a failure

In order to reduce the 'advantages' he was given access to a Walkman®, which was effective in giving him temporary relief from the voices, and the agreed alternative strategy for providing relief from stress and for getting attention from staff was that he would seek out staff to talk to them about how he was feeling. To reduce the long-term advantage of feeling that cutting his arms made him a more important patient, the advantages and disadvantages of people showing interest because of his disabilities rather than his abilities were discussed and he agreed that he would rather people were interested in him as a person than as a patient. There was general agreement within the staff team to take care to show special interest in what he was doing when he was well and to put more emphasis on his non-illness-related activities.

14

Modifying the delusional beliefs about the nature of the hallucinations

INTRODUCTION

Patients may be upset not only by what their voice says but also by who is saying it. Often this is what gives the voice such power and authority over the patient, so modifying his delusional beliefs about the nature of the voice can be a very important step in reducing its ability to distress.

Essentially the same approach is used to modify delusional ideas about voices as is used for other delusional ideas, so this chapter should be read as a sequel to Chapter 9. As with other delusional beliefs, you must set the goal for modification in order to be able to plan the most appropriate lines of therapy. The modification may be complete or partial and the goal should include not only what the patient will stop believing about the nature of the voice but also what new beliefs will stand in its stead. And, as with other delusional beliefs, although you will probably not be able to discuss the goal directly with your patient, you should indirectly check out how he would feel about the replacement belief (which is usually that the voice comes from within himself or from his own brain) to ensure that it will be more helpful and more welcome to him than his delusional one.

Some voices may be unpleasant in what they say but nevertheless the patient does not want to lose them because he does not want to lose the relationship with the source of the voice; this is most likely to occur when the source of the voice is important for religious reasons or when it is a close friend or family member. In these circumstances you should not go for a belief modification about the voice's origin unless there are compelling reasons for doing so; for example, the voice of God might be welcomed by the patient but if it were suggesting that he kill himself or others then this consideration would almost certainly outweigh the former when you were goal setting. If you want to affect the voice without affecting the patient's belief about its nature, then the practical strategies arc the safest option (see Chapter 10).

Some patients have pleasant and unpleasant voices coming from different identified sources. Where these two types of voice coexist it may not be possible to modify the patient's belief about the origin of the unpleasant voices without also affecting his belief about the pleasant ones. This being so, you should only proceed to attempt modification of the belief about the unpleasant voices if you are sure that your patient would gain overall even if his belief about the pleasant ones gets modified in the process. For example, with one of our patients who disliked hearing his neighbours criticising him but who was comforted by hearing his mother speaking words of encouragement when he was sad or lonely, it was decided not to attempt modification about the neighbours' voices for fear that this might destroy the ability of the pleasant voices to comfort him.

Delusional ideas about the source of a voice are often supported by the contcnt of that voice and vice versa, so these two lines of therapy are interlwined and normally proceed together. For example, proving that the voice cannot accurately predict the future would not only show that it cannot be believed when it predicts the patient's death in three years time but also that it could not be God talking: alternatively, proving that the voice was not from God would immediately take away its authority to predict the patient's future death. It is possible to work on the content of the voice without impinging on the delusional beliefs about its origin but, as we saw in Chapter 13, you have to be very careful if you wish to leave the delusional belief intact. For example, with a patient who is distressed by his mother's critical remarks but does not want to lose this contact with her, it may be possible to argue that the mother is only being critical because she does not understand his present circumstances or that she is only pretending to be critical for some reason, but whilst the patient continues to believe that it is his mother talking, the voice will continue to have power to distress.

MAKING THE GENERAL SPECIFIC

With hallucinations, making the general specific will apply not only to the delusional beliefs about the voice but also to its physical characteristics. Thcsc latter will include volume, clarity, direction, location, sex, accent and identity of each voice and, if there is more than one voice, whether the voices speak together or separately. When asked, patients are often unable to distinguish the sex or location of a voice, or to say whether there are one or more voices present, characteristics that would be easy to describe with a 'real' voice. If your patient is vague about his voice then you should accept and agree that it is somehow different from voices that come from other people, because you will be able to use this 'difference' later in therapy as evidence that the voices do not come from a physical source. Furthermore, once the patient is aware of a difference in physical characteristics then he may be able to learn to use this as a way of distinguishing his voices from the voices that come from real people (see Chapter 15, pp. 221–2).

LOGICAL REASONING

When asking questions about the voice, you should ask whether or not other people hear it. Most patients report readily that other people do not hear their voices: we have had a couple of patients who were surprised by the question, not having thought about it before, but we have never yet had a patient who believed that other people definitely could hear his voice. If your patient believes his voice comes from a real person then this is very obviously inconsistent with his belief that other people cannot hear it, but at this early stage you should not jump in to expose the inconsistency for fear of modifying the patient's belief about other people not being able to hear the voice; instead, you should be content to agree that the voice is 'somehow' different from ordinary voices and confirm that other people are unable to hear it.

Before exposing this inconsistency as part of the logical reasoning against the delusional belief, you should seek to establish that the voices of 'real' people can be heard by everyone in the same area. For example, you might discuss with your patient how we cannot voluntarily shut off our hearing (unlike our sight) so that if we are within earshot of two people talking we cannot avoid overhearing them, and anyone standing with us would also hear what was said. You can back up your patient's own experience of hearing everything that is going on in his vicinity by explaining to him why this is so, in terms of soundwaves coming from the mouth and expanding out to cover all areas of the room. Having established that if a real person is talking then other people in the hearer's vicinity must also be able to hear what he says, this can then be used as an argument against the patient's 'voice' coming from a real person.

As with other delusional beliefs, a good starting point in your attempts to detect other possible inconsistencies in your patient's belief about his voices is to ask yourself (i) why you do not believe as he does and (ii) how things would be different if the delusional belief were true. For example, one of our patients heard President Bush talking to him but if this were true then he would have been more likely to hear him during President Bush's daytime hours; in fact, the patient heard the President during his own daytime, i.e. when the President would have been asleep, so this was different from what one would expect if the delusion had been true. As with other delusions, your patient is likely to have some appreciation of the implication of his being unable to answer your questions about the voices or of inconsistencies in his answers, so direct questioning must be done sensitively and you should always be alert to back off.

Caution: Logical reasoning, backed up by reality testing if necessary, is very effective in countering delusional explanations about voices perceived to come from specific, real people, for example, the patient who believed he heard his parents who lived 20 miles away. Because it is so easy to prove the delusional belief wrong in these cases it is important not to rush in too quickly before the preparatory work has been done to ensure that the replacement belief is more acceptable. Coming in too soon will at best risk damaging rapport and at worse could push the patient into another, less easily challenged delusional explanation for his experiences. In the early stages of exposing an inconsistency it may be sufficient to note that the apparent inconsistency casts doubt on the patient's explanation being the 'whole' truth, without dwelling on the point, e.g. 'That doesn't seem to quite fit ... it's a bit of a puzzle, isn't it? But I don't suppose it really matters'.

EVIDENCE FOR AND AGAINST

As with other delusional beliefs, a key aspect of modifying delusional beliefs about voices is to find out from the patient what his belief is based on, what evidence he has to support it, and if he is aware of any evidence that seems to contradict it.

Voices that are attributed to people known to the patient are nearly always based on the evidence that the voice sounds the same as that person's. The approach in these cases is to use the argument that because the voice sounds as if it comes from that person does not mean that it *does* come from that person. If your patient has ever made mistakes in identifying voices of real people in the past then you can use this to back up this line of argument. You may also use the fact that we 'hear' people's voices in dreams even though they do not really come from the person concerned. If your patient has vivid auditory imagery, i.e. voices that he imagines sound very real to him, then it may be a useful exercise to get him to recall someone's voice or to imagine them talking during a therapy session, to show that 'hearing' (i.e. in imagination) is not the same as the person actually speaking, and furthermore that you can 'hear' them saying things that they would never say in real life.

Another important source of evidence that the patient has about the nature of the voice comes from what it says; this is particularly important where the voice is not recognised from its physical characteristics, for example, with a spirit voice. The voice may actually tell the patient who it is, or the patient may deduce who it is from what it is saying. In either case, the voice's utterances can be subjected to logical reasoning, evidence collection and reality testing, as described in Chapter 9, and the voice itself can be challenged in the various ways described in Chapter 13. If the only evidence to support the source of the voice is its own claim, then the therapeutic approach is to develop the argument that saying something does not guarantee that it is true. This can be developed as a general line of argument, referring to the frequent occasions when people in everyday life say things that are inaccurate or frankly untrue. Even better, if you can show that the voice has been wrong about anything that it has said in the past, then this provides more specific evidence that it could also be wrong or lying about who it claims to be. If the voice provides any other evidence to support its claim of who it is, then this would be challenged in the normal ways.

One line of argument that is peculiar to delusional ideas about voices is when there is an inconsistency between the content and origin of the voice, i.e. when what the voice says is atypical of what the person/ entity would actually say or might be expected to say. For example, one of our patients would hear people she knew and liked calling her abusive names even though they were always pleasant and polite to her in real life, so she was able to use this inconsistency as one piece of evidence to suggest that the voices did not come from the people they sounded like. Similarly, another patient was able to argue that his voice could not be coming from the Archangel Gabriel, who was understood to be a very 'good' spirit, because some of his criticisms were so harsh and unkind.

ALTERNATIVE EXPLANATIONS

Information coming from our senses is always very persuasive, presumably because normally it is a very reliable source of information about the external world, but unfortunately this means that hearing voices can also be very convincing. When the voice speaks the patient must disbelieve either the experience or the arguments and evidence collected during therapy. With the compelling evidence of the experience, he may discount the rational arguments and revert back to his delusional belief, at least whilst the voice is speaking. In order to counter this persuasive experience and the 'obvious' explanation for it, the patient must have a very good understanding of how the brain could produce a voice that sounds as real as it does and that says what it does. For this reason, it is important that the alternative explanation for his hallucinations is expressed in terms that make sense and are plausible to him (see Chapter 11, pp. 184–7).

REALITY TESTING

Where the voice is transmitted by soundwaves

It is easy to prove convincingly with reality testing that voices heard as coming from real people could not possibly be coming from them, so in these cases reality testing should be considered the final phase before belief modification takes place.

Reality testing whether the voice comes from real people is likely to include setting up situations for the patient to discover facts about real voices, so that he can discover the discrepancies between his voice and these voices. From your patient's detailed description of his voice, you will be aware of these potential discrepancies and therefore be able to set up the appropriate tests. For example, one of our patients heard his friend's voice from a house several miles away so we set up situations to show how far real voices carry. Other factors that are commonly explored in these tests are how the volume changes with distance (e.g. for the patient who discovered that his voice sounded just as loud however far he was from the person who seemed to be producing it), how intervening barriers like doors or buildings affect the sound (e.g. for the patient who could hear her voice coming from behind a large office block) and the fact that the patient can tell the sex, direction, etc. of real sounds (e.g. for the patient who could never tell whether his voice was a male or female and the patient who could never say where the voice was coming from). For these exercises, we usually ask two people that the patient trusts to walk up and down talking to one another or a single person to walk up and down reciting a list or poem. Both the patient and therapist note down when they can hear and when they cannot, what they hear and how clearly, and then they discuss their findings. Remember, because reality testing can disprove a delusional belief so dramatically, you must discuss the test and its interpretation with your patient before you carry it out.

I am always aware of the risk that proving the voice is not a physical sound might force the patient to explain his experience in terms of radio-waves or some more esoteric means of communication. This would be a highly undesirable belief change since this type of explanation is potentially much harder to disprove than the soundwave one. In practice, however, I have found that these alternatives do not arise providing you do not confront the patient with the reality test too soon, that is, before you have prepared him for the alternative belief about the voice coming from within. Nevertheless, as we saw in Chapter 9, it is always possible to misjudge these situations, so if such an undesirable belief change were to occur you should close it down immediately, i.e. you state that you do not believe that this alternative is possible, giving your reasons for coming to this conclusion (see pp. 164–7.

Where the voice is not transmitted by soundwaves

Some patients do not consider that their voices come via normal sound-waves even though they are thought to come from real people, whilst voices from alien or spirit forces nearly always come via radiowaves or some sort of telepathic communication. In these cases, reality testing to prove that the voice is not a real voice would be inappropriate and irrelevant.

You may find the following lines of argument useful if your patient is attributing his voice to radiowaves. The human brain is not set up to send or receive radio signals because if it were:

1. we could talk to one another without speaking out loud or using telephones;
2. we could pick up TV and radio programmes in our heads without requiring TV and radio sets;
3. other people would be able to hear the voice;
4. if the voice only occurred at a specific frequency, then we would have to have tuning devices in our heads;
5. like radiowaves, the voice reception would be affected by being indoors or outdoors;
6. radio and TV waves have to come from and be received by things that are made up from metals (I am not quite sure why this is so, fortunately I have never been asked to explain it, but no doubt an electronics book would have the answer) but our brains are made of squashy, non-metallic material.

Where the means of communication is some type of direct, telepathic link it is very much harder to challenge it. Apart from asking your patient and/or his voice how the communication works, and either noting that there is no apparent explanation or challenging the explanation given, the only thing you can do is to challenge the voice to communicate with you or other people and show that it cannot do that.

Directly challenging the voice to prove who it is

We saw in Chapter 13 how the voice could be disempowered by challenging it to harm the therapist. The voice can also be challenged to affect the therapist in other ways; for example, challenging the 'ghost' to inhabit the therapist or challenging the spirit who woke the patient at night to wake the therapist instead. Failure to meet these challenges weakens the perceived power of the voice and can also be used to cast doubt on its identity. Note that if the Walkman® or earplug affects the voice then this can be used similarly to disempower and cast doubt on the origin of the voice; for example, surely someone as powerful as the Archangel would be able to be heard above the Walkman when ordinary human beings, by talking loudly, can break through the music.

If your patient is willing to talk directly to his voice then the failure of the voice to respond appropriately to him is good evidence it is not coming from whom it claims to be coming. The first type of challenge is to ask the voice for information or knowledge that the 'owner' of the voice would have but that the patient does not have; for example, one of our patients asked the voice of John Lennon when he had been born. The second type of challenge is to ask the voice to do something that the 'owner' of the voice would be able to do; for example, one of our patients who could communicate with the Secret Service asked it to send him a letter through the post to confirm its instructions to stay in hospital.

CHECKING AND RECAPPING

As with other delusional beliefs, you should be sure to recap frequently and check that your understanding of the outcome and implications of your work is the same as your patient's. Rephrasing and re-evaluation is a continuous process that happens at all stages of therapy, but it is particularly important when new arguments are agreed, when new evidence comes in and when the alternative, replacement beliefs about the voices are developed.

Example from clinical practice

A young man had left university two years previously when he had been admitted to hospital with what he described as 'mental exhaustion'. He now lived in a flat on his own, which he liked, except for his complaint 'I wish my father would stop accusing me of being a failure: I know I am a failure, but it's upsetting when I'm sitting quietly or trying to get to sleep to hear him berating me'.

The goals of treatment were to modify his underlying belief that he was a failure, to control the voices and to modify his belief that the voice came from his father. The replacement belief was to be that the voice came from his own brain and was based on his memory of hurtful things that had been said to him by his father.

Work similar to that described in Chapter 8 (see p. 118) was undertaken to build up the patient's self-esteem, modifying the basis of his self-worth from academic and occupational achievements to personal factors. He found that he was able to temporarily stop the voices by using a Walkman so that sometimes he would be able to fall asleep with the Walkman still playing.

The way the patient talked about his symptoms indicated that he had no insight into their nature, and the use of the term 'mental exhaustion' strongly suggested that the notion of mental illness was not a welcome one, so a necessary preparatory stage before modifying the delusional belief about the origin of the voice was to destigmatise the notion of mental illness. The alternative explanation for his voices was prepared by discussing the occurrence of hallucinations in everyday life and as the result of illness.

Unfortunately, the content of the voices accurately reflected his father's opinion of the patient and so we could not use their unpleasantness as evidence that the voice did not come from his father. We were able to use the patient's own knowledge and experience of hearing sounds in different situations to reason that he would not be able to hear his father's voice from a house five miles away and so it was not necessary to conduct a formal reality test. One of the successful arguments we put forward was that if he could hear his father's voice clearly then he ought similarly to be able to hear at least 10 000 other voices who were in houses within the same five-mile radius as his parents' house.

In practice, the desired belief change about the origin of the voice occurred at this stage of the treatment. Although it was not necessary, the therapist had planned to suggest that the patient questioned the voice to determine whether it came from his father. Since the only source of information about the father was the patient himself it would not have been productive to question the voice about personal matters, but as his father was an accountant (which his son was not) it would have been possible to ask the voice about technical, accountancy matters.

Long-term strategies for delusions and hallucinations

15

INTRODUCTION

In planning long-term strategies for delusions and hallucinations, one assumes that the delusional ideas and experiences may continue to bother the patient from time to time, either because they are not adequately controlled by the medication or because there is a relapse in the illness. The essence of long-term therapy is for the patient to be able to identify his symptoms when they occur, so that he can put into effect measures to counter them. Long-term strategies include the CBT strategies found to be most effective during therapy together with coping strategy enhancement and relapse prevention work. Where medication has proved beneficial, the key aspect of the long-term work may be CBT to improve medication compliance (see Chapter 16).

ENCOURAGE RECOGNITION AND LABELLING OF SYMPTOMS

After a degree of insight has been achieved during therapy, many patients spontaneously start to label their delusions and hallucinations (e.g. 'It's one of my odd ideas', 'It's just a voice'). This is a very positive step forward because it helps the patient discriminate more clearly between what is due to his illness and what is not. Not only does this help to reduce the impact of the thoughts or voices (e.g. 'If it's only one of my paranoid ideas then that means that X isn't really trying to poison me'), it also provides the patient with a clear focus and trigger for learn cognitive and other coping strategies to be applied (e.g. 'If it's one of my paranoid ideas I will feel better if I leave my room and go to talk to someone'). Whilst some labels may stem from the therapist and be mutually agreed during rephrasing and recapping, wherever possible it is better to use the patient's own words for labelling as these are likely to be more accurate in describing his own experiences.

During therapy, you and your patient may have identified certain characteristic features of his delusional ideas and hallucinations, for example, they might relate to a particular person or be triggered by illicit drug use. These characteristics can be noted down for use as a checklist to help the patient detect the delusional ideas and hallucinations when they occur. Note that 'detection' does not necessarily mean that the patient is immediately able to recognise the idea as *definitely* delusional or to recognise that what he hears is *definitely* an hallucination; often the goal is for the patient to recognise that this *could* be a delusional idea or hallucination and therefore that he should apply the various tests and techniques learned during therapy in order to examine it further.

Delusions

It is not easy to detect delusional ideas in oneself but the following characteristics may be useful.

The content of a specific delusion

Where delusional beliefs are quite specific and recur in this same specific form, they are potentially easier for the patient to detect as delusional than vague, general ideas because the patient knows exactly what to look out for. For example, 'I know that one of my paranoid ideas is that my brother is trying to poison me, so if I get this idea then it is a sign that my illness is having a dip again; my brother doesn't want to poison me and I know this because...'.

A particular theme of the delusions

In some patients, recurring delusional ideas may involve the same theme but have a different focus, for example, when different people become targets of a paranoid feeling. In this case, the patient may learn to be sensitive and alert for particular themes in his ideas; for example, 'I know that I can develop paranoid ideas about people, so if I get a feeling that someone wants to harm me this could be one of those paranoid ideas. I must look for objective evidence that would be acceptable in a court of law to back up the feeling, and I might be able to check it out by.... If I can't find any evidence to prove the feeling then I will know it is one of my paranoid ideas and not true.'

Other features associated with the occurrence of delusional ideas

Patients may be able to use other features of their illness to alert themselves to the fact that they will be particularly susceptible to delusional beliefs at this time and therefore should be particularly careful to check out any potentially delusional ideas. For example, one of our patients who experienced a sense of 'life speeding up' when he became unwell was able to incorporate this into his coping strategies. Whenever he got this feeling he would rigorously check all ideas he had about people being against him by looking for evidence and asking friends what they thought.

Hallucinations can be a useful indicator of worsening psychosis because they are easier for the patient to detect than delusional ideas; for example, one patient developed the strategy 'If I can hear those voices again I must be careful because at these times I am very likely to get the idea that someone is trying to harm me in some way. These feelings are very convincing but when I have checked them out in the past they have proved not to be true in fact, so although the feeling may be very persuasive now I must look for proof to back it up. If I can't find any proof this means it is my brain misleading me and the person doesn't really wish me any harm'. Another patient learned to be particularly vigilant for the first couple of hours after getting out of bed in the morning: 'I very often get horrible thoughts about the staff interfering with me in the morning, but it goes by lunchtime and in the afternoon I realise that they like me and wouldn't want to harm me'.

Other commonly reported associated features are sleeping poorly, feeling agitated/stressed and problems with thinking.

Hallucinations

One or more of the following criteria may be useful in helping the patient to recognise when one of his 'voices' has occurred.

The physical characteristics of the voice (e.g. sex, direction, distance, volume)

If the patient is able to detect something different about his hallucinatory voices then this can help him to decide whether or not a 'voice' has been heard; for example, 'If I can't tell which direction it's coming from, then it must be one of my voices' or 'If it sounds as if it's coming from just 2–3 inches away, then that's being produced by my own brain'.

In some cases the patient may learn to recognise that there is something different about a 'voice', or some different sort of feeling associated with hearing it, even though he is not able to describe this in words. He should be encouraged to recognise this 'difference' when it occurs. For example, with one of our patients we found that when she heard her hallucinatory voice she was only 95% certain that it came from a real person, whereas with a real person she was 100% certain. Having identified this feature, she was able to use the check 'If I'm only 95% certain it's real then it's not, it's one of my voices'.

The particular words used

Some patients' voices say essentially the same thing, in the same words, even though different voices may be heard saying them. When this occurs it is very helpful for long-term therapy because detailing the typical remarks of the voices provides the patient with an easy way of checking what he hears. For example, one patient's voices always said 'You're a hypocrite' or 'You're talking through your hat' so he learned that whenever he heard these accusations they were voices and not coming from real people. In other cases, the words used may be atypical of the people they seem to be coming from, for example, when obscene words seem to be coming from strangers or lewd remarks are heard during a social conversation, and this can be used to recognise that a 'voice' has occurred.

In some cases the hallucinations tend to include particular words or phrases and so, once these have been detected, the patient can use them to identify a 'voice'. For example, one of our patients noted that his voice was particularly likely to use the words 'well, actually' whilst another discovered that being addressed as 'bitch' was typical of the voice but atypical of everyday social contacts.

A particular theme of the voices

Voices typically follow certain specific themes for individual patients, for example, sexual history, sins committed in the past, envy, etc. Once these themes have been identified they can be used by the patient as an alert to the possibility or even probability that it came from a 'voice'. For example, he might be able to reason. 'Be careful, this is the sort of thing my voice says, I need to check where it's coming from before I act on it' or it might trigger him to bring other checking mechanisms into play, like asking a friend if he had heard the voice too, or asking himself if it is likely that the person concerned would have said what he apparently heard him say.

DEVELOP SETS OF ARGUMENTS AND CHALLENGES TO COUNTER SPECIFIC DELUSIONS AND HALLUCINATIONS

Practical experience has shown that in times of relapse it is the same delusional beliefs that tend to recur, even if they are disavowed in between (see Chapter 2). This being so, it is possible to collect together the logical arguments, evidence and reality-testing results that were found to be useful during therapy so that they can be used immediately to combat the re-emerging delusion and prevent it becoming firmly established. Similarly, you should take your patient through the most effective challenges to his voices as many times as necessary to ensure that they come to him naturally and spontaneously whenever the voice occurs.

DEVELOP/ENHANCE COPING STRATEGIES

Develop coping statements

Coping statements are peculiar to each individual patient, being built up from the rational arguments and evidence obtained about the delusions; for example, 'The voice has lied in the past, so I shouldn't believe it now' and 'I know from the experiments we did that no-one else can hear the voice, so I don't have to get off the train to ensure that other people won't hear it'. Coping statements are often used to trigger coping behaviours; for example, 'If I am beginning to feel isolated in my room I am particularly likely to get the feeling that people don't like me any more, but I have found in the past that going down to the day centre helps stop that feeling. So although it feels like a tremendous effort, I must make that effort and go to the day centre; it will be well worth it in the long run. I will treat myself to a cake when I get home.'

Coping during 'bad patches'

Fluctuations in psychosis are common in the medication-resistant population and often, when in relapse, patients feel as if they have always felt this bad and that it will never get any better. In these circumstances, it may be comforting as well as helpful for the patient to develop a coping statement around the duration of these fluctuations or 'bad patches'. Going through the past case notes and carefully monitoring these periods as they occur during therapy will enable you and your patient to write a statement in the form of 'Although I feel as if this will go on for ever, in the past it has usually lasted for about ... days, so if I can just keep going it *will* get better'. Insight into the nature and likely extent of a 'bad patch' may also help to prevent dysfunctional behaviour, the more extreme forms of which can include violence to self or others. For example, one of our patients who put her arm through windows when she felt bad developed a statement, 'If I can just keep going for another couple of days without putting my arm through a window I *will* feel better then and be able to enjoy myself again, but if I have put my arm through a window I may be transferred to the locked ward and then I won't be able to ride my bicycle. If I feel really tense I can go into the garden and shout at the roses'.

Develop a set of practical coping behaviours

Like other people, people with schizophrenia can usually affect how they feel to some extent by what they do, so behavioural coping strategies have a role to play alongside the cognitive ones. Even when the patient has good insight and can recognise a delusional idea or hallucination for what it is, when the psychosis is active he will still experience the unpleasant emotions associated with the symptoms (see Chapter 2) so these practical strategies can be an important feature for long-term CBT. Practical strategies are not targeted directly at the delusion or hallucination but aim to lessen the impact by indirect means, usually through distraction and/or by reducing stress/arousal levels. The last three strategies described for hallucinations in Chapter 10 (pp. 176–7) are also appropriate for delusions.

Your patient may already have discovered for himself that acting in a particular way helps him to cope when he gets the unpleasant ideas and feelings, but he may not be using this in the most reliable or effective way. If this is the case you may be able to help him develop this strategy so that he uses it to maximal effect (so-called 'coping strategy enhancement'). To give a very simple example, a patient may report that he feels less paranoid if he gets out of his room every day and talks to other people, but nevertheless he remains isolated in his room for days on end because he has nowhere to go. Arranging for him to go to a day centre or putting him in touch with his local drop-in centre may be enough to enable him to put his 'going out' coping strategy into effect when he needs to. You can also tell your patient about strategies that other people have found effective and suggest that he might like to try some of these to see if they are helpful for him.

One of the advantages of practical coping strategies is that they can often be used by the patient even if he has no insight about his illness or the symptoms, so they can be used before the cognitive strategies are in place or when the psychosis relapses so badly that insight is lost and the cognitive strategies are no longer applied.

Relapse prevention and medication/treatment compliance

Early detection of relapse enables appropriate action to be taken before the effects of the psychosis become overwhelming. Therefore, an important set of coping strategies to develop is concerned with the detection and response to early signs of relapse. A list of warning signs can be built up when the patient is relatively well and written down for him to use, either at regular intervals, as a sort of checklist, or when he begins to feel unwell. Since hallucinations are generally easier to detect than delusions the re-emergence of hallucinations may be an important early indicator of worsening psychosis. Where appropriate, it is useful for the carer to have a similar (it is unlikely to be identical) set of warning signs, also written down.

Once the possibility of relapse is detected, the patient refers to his 'action plan' for what to do. These actions may include items such as 'Phone the CPN' or 'Tell my carer' or more idiosyncratic items such as 'Cut down on the alcohol' or 'Don't stay indoors on your own'. Since the patient may not be able to detect relapse in himself and may even be antagonistic towards any intervention at this time, there should also be an agreed plan of action for the carer to take should certain signs or criteria be met, for example, for the carer to contact the doctor or social worker if the patient starts to hear gunfire from outside his house. The advantage of having agreed and formally recorded this action *before* the patient becomes unwell is that it helps the carer to counter any accusation of betrayal (e.g. 'You asked me to contact your CPN if ... '); this may not be very effective at the time but it may help to repair the trusting relationship later.

Having the warning signs of worsening illness identified and written down not only alerts the patient to the possibility of a relapse when this occurs but also has the less obvious benefit of helping the patient and carer *not* to immediately attribute everything unusual to worsening of the illness, for example, an outburst of temper or not sleeping one night.

Where medication is beneficial in keeping the patient's psychosis under control, CBT may be useful for improving medication compliance: indeed, medication is such an important coping strategy for some patients that improving compliance may be the most important goal for the CBT (see Chapter 16).

MAKE CARDS OF THE EFFECTIVE CBT STRATEGIES

One of the key elements for the success of long-term strategies is to ensure that your patient puts the measures into effect when he needs to do so. When under the compelling influence of a delusional idea or hallucinatory voice, he may find it hard to recall the lines of logical reasoning you used in therapy or the disconfirming evidence that was collected. Whilst sitting with you in your office may be a sufficient trigger to set the CBT strategies into motion, they may not occur to him when he is sitting on his own in his hostel with his voices nagging away at him or with the overwhelming conviction that his ideas are true. In order for your patient to have ready access to the most effective strategies even when he is on his own, you should summarise the lines of argument, evidence, results of reality tests, coping behaviours, etc. on cards which he can carry with him (see examples below). Note that this is normally done as a joint exercise, so the card contains the things that the patient has found to be persuasive and helpful, and these are expressed in his own words.

We have found from experience that the cards should be small enough to be kept in handbags or pockets and strong enough to withstand being crushed against other things; A5 card or file cards are convenient. You should keep photocopies of the cards in your notes, not only for the sake of having an accurate record but also in case the patient loses his copy and urgently requires another.

The use of audio tapes would seem to have potential in this area, since one might expect that hearing the arguments actually used during a session might be even stronger than seeing them written down. None of our patients has ever wanted this in practice, but it is worth asking your patient if you think he might be interested in having the therapy reinforced in this way.

Examples from clinical practice

Note: Whether the cards are written in terms of 'I' or 'You' is a matter of personal preference and differs from patient to patient.

Patient 1
The following card was developed for a female patient who heard voices of unknown origin, usually accusing her of something which was actually false or instructing her to do something to harm herself. The card incorporates the particular strategies that she had found helpful. Note that, in her case, directly questioning the voice always shut it up for a while, so it was a safe and effective strategy to use.

CHALLENGING THE VOICES

To get rid of the voice
1. Tell the voice that you know it tells lies and talks nonsense.
2. Tell the voice to go away.
3. Use a Walkman® to stop the voice.
4. Go and talk to someone.
5. Go on a brisk walk.
6. Avoid TV, because you may get false 'messages' from it.

To challenge the voice
1. Ask it for EVIDENCE to support its claims, e.g. when the voice is accusing you or other people of something.
2. Go through your individual cards if you need to remind yourself of the evidence AGAINST what the voice is saying.
3. If a voice tells you to do something, ask 'WHY SHOULD I?'. Tell the voice 'I don't trust you – you've told me to do some terrible things in the past, e.g. drink poison – you've never told me anything that's for my good'.
4. If the voice says you are responsible for some event, ask 'HOW COULD I BE RESPONSIBLE FOR THAT?'.

Patient 2
The example given below is of a card used by a lady who had recurrent feelings that people hated her.

When I get the feeling that people hate and despise me that's due to my brain chemistry. Therefore, other people do not really hate me, even though I feel that they do.

Evidence that the feeling is due to my brain chemistry
1. It wouldn't make sense that people would change so drastically from day to day about how they felt about me when nothing has happened between us. For example, when I kept a record I noted that it felt as if Maureen hated me on days 3 and 5 but on the other days I knew that she liked me.
2. There would be no reason for people who knew nothing about me to hate me.
3. The feelings are worse before my period is due.
4. Whenever I've actually asked people if they hate me they've told me they don't.
5. When I look for evidence that my friends and family hate me I can never find anything that would stand up in a court of law. Actually they continue to do nice things even when I feel they hate me.
6. The only reason I have to think people hate me is the strong intuitive feeling that I get, but even very strong feelings can be quite wrong.

When I get the feeling that people hate me
1. When I get the feeling that people hate me it's my brain being oversensitive and giving me the wrong message. My higher

thinking is better able to work things out and tell me what is really happening, so I should rely on what my reasoning tells me, not the intuitional feelings.

2. These feelings only last for a day or at most two, so if I can stop myself being snappy with people I won't upset them and have to apologise later.

3. Sometimes I feel better if I go off to my room and listen to my music.

4. Also, if I talk to staff about what I feel they can remind me that this is only a feeling, that it won't last and that people really like me.

INTRODUCTION

For nearly all people with schizophrenia, antipsychotic medication offers the best chance of gaining relief from their symptoms. Although there are undoubtedly a few patients who seem to get no benefit at all from the drugs currently available, and a few more for whom the unpleasant side effects outweigh the benefits, the range of antipsychotic drugs now available is such that very few patients get no benefit at all from medication and so taking the medication prescribed is, for the large majority of patients, their most important coping strategy. However, if a patient has little or no insight into his illness it is quite reasonable from his point of view to consider medication inappropriate, and if he is aware of unpleasant side effects or, as sometimes happens, actually blames the medication for his psychotic symptoms, then it is understandable if he is unwilling to take it.

ETHICAL CONSIDERATIONS

A patient may be non-compliant for two broad reasons: either he does not want to take the medication or he wants to take it but forgets or fails to do so for other reasons. Where the patient wants to be compliant there are no ethical issues with medication compliance work because, as the therapist, you are following the basic principle of using CBT to help the patient achieve his own goals. However, where the patient does not want to take the medication prescribed, and will very likely have expressed this explicitly as well as implying it by his behaviour, you are faced with an immediate ethical problem – should you embark on a course of 'therapy' where your goal is diametrically opposed to that of your patient, especially as you will probably have to keep your goal concealed from your patient at the start of therapy?

Whilst the resolution of this ethical dilemma will rest on consideration of each individual case, we have found it helpful to consider that our primary aim with people referred for poor medication compliance is not improved medication compliance *per se* but rather to improve the patient's sense of well-being, which may (or may not) be achieved through medication compliance. With this approach you can have an agreed goal (implicit or explicit) with your patient, namely of trying to find something that would improve things for him in some way. This is genuine and honest on your part but avoids the likely conflict and loss of rapport if you were to immediately broach the medication issue. Of course, this approach does mean that you should keep an open mind about whether or not medication has an overall beneficial result for your patient and not just assume that it is a good thing because your colleague has prescribed it.

ENGAGEMENT AND RAPPORT

An obvious but necessary prerequisite for medication compliance therapy to be successful is that your patient attends the therapy sessions, but by the very nature of this patient population, engagement in treatment programmes is problematic. At best, patients are likely to be indifferent to the prospect of meeting regularly with you and at worst they may be actively hostile to the idea of seeing someone associated with the mental health team or to talking about the unpleasant treatment for an illness that they do not have. More than with any other aspect of CBT with schizophrenia, in this area of work you will need to be both flexible and very tolerant with respect to appointments and your patient's attendance.

If you can meet your patient fairly informally, before starting the CBT, this may be helpful in demonstrating that you are friendly and non-threatening. If your patient has a history of revolving-door admissions then it may be easier to get to know him and to start working with him whilst he is an inpatient, with the hope that you will have built up a sufficiently strong relationship for him to want to continue to see you after discharge. But in any case, you must expect most of the effort and inconvenience of meeting together to come from you and not from the patient: after all, since he sees no potential benefits in meeting with you it would be unreasonable to expect him to put himself out to keep your appointments.

PROVIDING A RATIONALE FOR TAKING MEDICATION

Typically, non-compliers deny that they have an illness, so a common goal is to promote understanding of their symptoms in terms of some biochemical abnormality that can be corrected by medication. If this implies that they have an illness/schizophrenia then care must be taken to destigmatise these concepts before the insight is pursued.

If the patient is resistant to the notion of illness, then it is not necessary to go for this particular insight to achieve compliance. Medication can be as relevant for helping symptoms attributed to LSD, x-rays, ghosts, etc. as for symptoms attributed to illness/schizophrenia.

CBT WITH SYMPTOMS/ISSUES THAT CONCERN THE PATIENT

As a general rule, it is advisable not to concentrate on medication issues in the early stages of therapy. Following the medication agenda may at best be interpreted by the patient as showing lack of understanding and concern for his 'real' problems and at worst as showing that you are part of the 'establishment' who are only interested in getting him to take (undesirable) medication. You should build up rapport by concentrating on issues that concern your patient and by trying to help with these, using CBT or other psychosocial techniques as appropriate.

In applying the CBT approach to any disturbing delusions or hallucinations, the patient's insight and understanding about the illness that underlies them are likely to be improved, opening a way for discussion of medication issues. Alternative explanations for his psychotic experiences in terms of his brain not functioning accurately are particularly useful in this respect.

MAKING THE CONNECTION BETWEEN 'BEING RELATIVELY WELL' AND 'ON MEDICATION'

Recall of what it was like on and off medication

Insight may be hampered, particularly in patients who are well at interview, by the patient's inability to recall what he was like, how he felt and how he acted when he was unwell. Since you may want to work with the patient to make the connection between being 'unwell' and 'off drugs' as compared to 'relatively well' and 'on drugs', it is important that he has access to this information about when he was unwell. If he is unable to recall his feelings or actions from those times you may (gently) tell him about the information in his medical record or, with his permission, seek the information from relatives or friends who knew him at that time. Your patient may not accept these versions of events but it does give you a good starting ground for discussing what might have gone on. Alternatively, if there is a risk that by merely reporting what others say you will be judged by your patient to be 'one of them', then you can encourage him to ask his doctor or other relevant person about these issues; this also has the advantage of giving him control of what and how much of this information is fed back to you both for discussion.

One of the major factors that hinders a patient making the connection between being off medication and worsening symptoms is the length of time between the last dose being taken and the illness relapse, a period that can extend to weeks where medication was in the form of depot injection. On first stopping medication, patients may actually notice an improvement in their general feeling of well-being because some of the side effects of the medication, for example drowsiness, may clear up quite quickly and so this tends to reinforce the belief that it was the medication that was making them feel unwell in the first place. It is perhaps not surprising that patients do not causally connect events that are separated by days or weeks since in everyday life substances taken by mouth or by injection tend to have much more rapid onset and short-lived effects, as for example with aspirin or alcohol. Education about how the medication works and, in particular, how long it stays in the body will be necessary before the patient can understand why something he did several weeks ago can make him feel poorly now, especially if he has felt better in between.

Showing that a connection could exist between missed medication and illness recurrence is particularly difficult where the patient has stayed well for weeks or even months after discontinuing medication. In this case you would have to explain the notion of a fluctuating illness and the role that medication plays in countering the adverse effects of the illness as and when they re-emerge, and in preventing their developing.

The relationship between 'medication' and 'feeling better'

The rationale for using the medication may range from the purely pragmatic, e.g. 'You seem to feel better when you're taking it than when you're not' to the causative, biochemical explanations, which may be given at different levels of sophistication according to the patient's ability to understand. Intermediate between these positions is to explain the beneficial effects in terms of some intermediary state, for example, that the medication helps the patient to get a better night's sleep or to feel less agitated, and that this is what makes the patient less sensitive to his evil spirits or enables him to ignore the voice of his neighbour. Similar partial explanations imply that changing the biochemistry of the patient's brain somehow makes him more resistant to the unpleasant happenings, for example, that the medication alters the biochemistry of the brain so that it becomes like other people's and can no longer be invaded by the ghost or hear the messages sent by the aliens. These intermediate positions do not challenge the underlying delusional beliefs but nevertheless assert that the beneficial effects are due to biological changes in the brain.

You should seek to discover, through discussion, what rationale makes most sense to your patient and to work with this, developing it if necessary, rather than starting off with the intention of imposing your own rationale.

EDUCATION ABOUT MEDICATION

Patients should be given information about their prescribed drugs, including side effects, according to their level of insight and understanding. Not only does the patient have a natural right to this information but also understanding how his medication works may help him to understand why he needs to take it. However, in telling the patient how his medication works you will be implying very directly that his experiences/beliefs are manifestations of a mental illness caused by a biochemical abnormality, and it is difficult not to imply that you consider medication to be a 'good thing'. If it is important for you to maintain your stance of neutral, collaborative enquiry regarding the effects of medication, then another member of the team should take the lead on the education work. Alternatively, there are now some excellent leaflets available, e.g. from The National Schizophrenia Fellowship and The Royal College of Psychiatrists, that describe how the different medications work. A secondary advantage of you not being the one to explain about the medication effects is that by asking your patient about what he has been told or read, you will be able to assess how accurately he has understood the information and his attitude towards it.

The education about his medication needs to explain to the patient why he has to continue to take it even when he is apparently well. The analogy of diabetes can be a useful one to explain not only how medication may help to correct a chemical imbalance but also why it is necessary to continue to take it in order to remain well.

For patients who can stay well for months at a time without medication, in between acute relapses, education should include the emerging evidence from clinical trials that patients do better in the long term if they can avoid having acute relapses, and so regular medication is likely to be preferable even though they would have periods when they would be symptom free without.

MODIFICATION OF DYSFUNCTIONAL BELIEFS ABOUT MEDICATION

Asking the patient what it is like to be on medication may reveal not only the side effects that he experiences but also any dysfunctional or delusional beliefs he may have about the medication or the side effects;

these may be about taking medicine in general (e.g. 'It's a sign of weakness to take pills') or about the patient's particular medicine (e.g. 'It makes my muscles weak' or 'It's damaging my heart'). Where dysfunctional beliefs exist they should be tackled by CBT and/or education.

Some patients are reluctant to take maintenance medication on the grounds that this implies that they are still ill, or that taking medication implies that they are not normal. A counter for this dysfunctional belief is to explain that the medication corrects the patient's biochemistry so he is 'well' or 'normal', i.e. his biochemistry is like that of other people, when he is taking the medication, and only 'ill' or 'abnormal' when he is not. The analogy of diabetes can be useful to illustrate this point.

A particularly difficult obstacle to compliance is when the patient attributes his residual psychotic symptoms to his medication, for example, 'It's the chlorpromazine that's making my thoughts muddled' or 'It's the drugs that make me hear voices, I was fine before'. If the patient's recall of his becoming ill is vague and confused, which it may very well be, it is not surprising if he associates the symptoms with the medication, since they both started at roughly the same time. This connection may be reinforced by the valid relationship that exists between the medication and some of his new experiences, for example if the medication has given him akathisia or feelings of being damped down. In order to show that the medication is reducing rather than creating the symptoms, you need to establish that your patient was more unwell before taking the medication (see above). If medication was only given after your patient was hospitalised, which is likely, then you can use the fact of the hospital admission to suggest/indicate that he must have been unwell before this, e.g. 'Would you have been brought into hospital if you were completely well?' or 'It costs a lot of money to keep people in hospital. What made people think that you needed it?'.

The most direct and probably convincing reality test of the effectiveness of medication would be to discontinue the medication and record the results. Although psychiatric staff are unlikely to set up such an experiment, it is not uncommon for the patient to effectively set it up himself by stopping taking the medication, in which case the opportunity should be taken to note what happens for later discussion.

ROLE OF PRESCRIBING DOCTOR AS 'TRUSTED EXPERT'

Treatment compliance is likely to be affected by the patient's perception and beliefs about the person prescribing it. To take two extreme examples, the patient with no insight about his illness and medication may continue to take his prescribed medication if he believes his doctor to be a knowledgeable, trustworthy and authoritative person who has the patient's best interest at heart, whereas a patient with good insight may nevertheless refuse medication if he believes his doctor to be useless or fears he wishes to do him harm. If treatment compliance is being adversely affected by dysfunctional beliefs about those prescribing or delivering the treatment, then it may be achieved by using CBT techniques to modify these beliefs. The first goal of modification is usually toward a belief that the prescribing doctor is genuinely trying to be helpful and has the patient's best interests at heart, even if his efforts are misguided and unsuccessful. In this cost-conscious age, a line of reasoning that may be persuasive is that the NHS would not 'waste' £x (whatever the cost of the patient's medication, hospital admission, CPN visits, etc.) unless it felt it was really necessary.

THE ADVANTAGES AND DISADVANTAGES OF TAKING THE PRESCRIBED MEDICATION (COST/BENEFIT ANALYSIS)

If your patient has no insight into being ill and if it is not possible or not desirable to promote this understanding, then your only way of securing voluntary medication compliance is if he recognises that he is in some way better when taking it than when not. Even when there is insight, at the end of the day a patient will only take medication if, for him, the perceived advantages outweigh the perceived disadvantages. This balance becomes particularly important when control of medication is entirely in the patient's own hands and there is no social or other pressure, e.g. role expectation as a patient in hospital, to encourage compliance.

From an early stage you should seek to build up an understanding of what the patient sees to be the advantages and disadvantages of taking his medication. One way of obtaining this information is to ask him why he takes his medication when he does and also why he stops taking it. The aim of medication compliance therapy is to decrease the perceived disadvantages of taking medication and increase the perceived advantages until that the balance is firmly in favour of the advantages. You should be sure to collect as many of the disadvantages of taking medication as possible, because you will not be able to reduce any disadvantages that you are not aware of. Any perceived disadvantages that are based on delusional or dysfunctional beliefs, e.g. 'The drugs turn my skin yellow' or 'People look down on me for taking drugs' or 'The medication makes me feel paranoid' should be modified using CBT principles, so that the patient can then discredit and discount them. Other disadvantages may be valid, in which case it may be possible to reduce them by practical means; for example, the patient who disliked having a 40-minute walk through the rain to get his depot injection was given these injections at home. Be careful not to minimise the unpleasantness of the side effects of some of these medications as they can be a very real deterrent to compliance. Apart from the side effects that patients can describe, e.g. restlessness and slow thinking, antipsychotic medication seems to have some very unpleasant effects that patients find very difficult to put into words but that make them reluctant to take it despite appreciating some of the advantages of doing so.

At the same time as reducing the disadvantages of medication, you should be developing the advantages by helping the patient to be more aware of and to understand the beneficial effects of the medication for him (see above). At some stage it may be helpful to formally record the 'advantages' and 'disadvantages' to help your patient weigh them up.

There are likely to be disadvantages associated both with being on and being off medication, so at the end of the day your patient will probably have to choose between the lesser of two evils. You may need to work specifically on this point, to help your patient see that, sadly, unlike other people, what is not possible is for him to be both well and free from the adverse effects of medication.

Note: If this work suggests to you either that the patient is getting no benefit from his medication or that the benefits are outweighed by the side effects, then you should report this finding back to the team and to the prescribing doctor in particular. It may be that a change of medication is indicated or even that the patient would be better on no medication at all. Remember, your role is only to improve compliance if that would be experienced by the patient as beneficial.

DEVELOPING GOOD HABITS FOR MEDICATION COMPLIANCE

Not all patients who fail to comply with medication do so because they believe it to be bad for them or even that they would be better off without it. In some cases patients may fail to take their medication, at least in the first instance, for practical reasons, for example, because they forget or because it is not convenient to go for their depot, etc. This being so, once your patient has decided that, on balance, he is better on medication than off it, you should work out with him the best possible regime to ensure that he does actually take the medication as prescribed. This may involve discussing practical arrangements (e.g. location of depot clinic, days of appointment, etc.) and making appropriate changes around those where possible. If the patient is forgetful or disorganised it may be more fruitful to ask others to make the changes rather than relying on the patient to do so, for example, asking staff at the depot clinic to phone the patient on the morning of his injection rather than trying to train him up in the use of a diary.

As anyone who has been on a course of antibiotics knows, it is surprisingly easy to forget to take medication, so it is important for the patient to develop a routine for taking his medication. Helping the patient develop an appropriate routine may be an important step in establishing compliance. The simpler and more repetitive the routine, the better chance it has of being established as a habit. The other important factor is to establish a trigger or prompt which will remind the patient to take his medication. For example, if your patient takes his pills at night and in the morning, it might be effective for him to leave his medication bottle next to his bedside cabinet, or if he brushes his teeth regularly twice a day, next to his toothbrush holder. Similarly, if the pills have to be taken at mealtimes and your patient takes sugar in his tea, then it might be effective for him to leave a reminder in his sugar bowl to take his medication. Dosset boxes (which, if necessary, can be filled by someone else) help to simplify more complicated drug regimes and provide an immediate reminder if a dose has been missed. Various electronic aids have been developed that can be useful for medication compliance, for example, the pill box that bleeps at regular intervals or the appointments reminder that can be set to ring at specific times during the day. Whatever the reminder chosen and routine developed, it must be one that fits in with the patient's general habits and lifestyle. If patients live at home or in a hostel, they may wish to include their relative or carer in their medication compliance routine, for example, by asking them to give a reminder when medication is due.

LONG-TERM COMPLIANCE WORK

If there is no agreement to take medication, or if at any stage during therapy your patient decides to stop taking it, then you can use this as an opportunity to record what happens with a view to presenting this as 'evidence' for his future consideration. As far as possible you would do this in collaboration with your patient, and ideally he would be doing some of the recording (though in practice this latter is often not possible, due to lost insight). Where patients have a revolving-door history of non-compliance, it may take several cycles of admission + medication → discharge → stop medication → relapse → admission to build up the evidence necessary for the patient to see the connection between coming off medication and re-emergence of symptoms. This requires both time and patience but it may be the only effective, albeit long-term, strategy to break the non-compliance cycle.

Appendix 1
Putting the therapy into practice, safely

This book was written in response to the demand for a practice manual from people attending our workshops and supervision sessions and is based on the feedback and follow-up from people attending our CBT with Schizophrenia courses, which are run through the Association of Psychological Therapies (P.O. Box 3, Thurnby, Leicester LE7 9QN) and the psychology department of our Specialist Services Unit. Our experience from the training courses is that although practising CBT therapists (mainly clinical psychologists) are most easily able to incorporate the new techniques into their existing ways of working, people from other professions and disciplines can and do develop into effective therapists, though they may be more unsure of themselves and need more practice to feel confident using the new approach. The overwhelming reaction from participants at the end of a course is one of enthusiasm to try to put what they have learned into practice with their own patients, and this they are encouraged to do.

As you will be well aware by this stage, this therapeutic approach is a very complex one, and some people are daunted by this. For this reason, it is recommended that you make frequent reference to the overall summary charts given in Appendix 2 when planning and carrying out the therapy. Whilst this is certainly not the only way of structuring this therapeutic approach, it has been found to be useful in reminding the therapist of the different possible strategies that could be used, the reason for doing them and how these relate and interact with one another.

In your early days as a therapist it is likely that you will not think of all the possible approaches that could be tried (this is often true for more experienced therapists, too) but it is better to try some potentially beneficial techniques than none at all, providing you apply these techniques safely. Some new therapists are worried that by discussing the delusional beliefs and voices with their patient, or in attempting to intervene, they may inadvertently make things worse. Whilst you certainly should not be gung-ho in your approach to this work, neither should your apprehension about making a possible mistake prevent you from trying these strategies with your patient. No doubt an unscrupulous therapist could make a patient's symptoms worse by misapplying CBT strategies, but he would need to set about this deliberately and, furthermore, have the expertise to know how to do it. Providing you are sensitive to your patient as a fellow human being it is highly unlikely that you will make things significantly worse for him by using CBT inexpertly; the worst thing to happen will be that your efforts will be ineffective, not that they will do any positive harm.

THE ESSENTIALS OF SAFE PRACTICE

1. **Set the goals of treatment and plan the possible lines of approach** *before* **making any attempt to challenge or modify a delusion or hallucination.**
2. **Prepare the alternative explanation** *before* **starting to challenge or modify the delusion or hallucination.**
   (a) Delusional beliefs make sense to the patient because they explain something. If the delusional belief is successfully challenged without a planned alternative being available to take its place then the patient will form his own alternative explanation to account for the 'something' that was previously explained by the delusion and there is a risk that this might also be delusional.
   (b) You must ensure that the alternative explanation is more acceptable and more functional for the patient than his delusional one. Where the alternative explanation is in terms of 'illness' or 'schizophrenia' you may need to destigmatise and normalise these explanations to ensure their acceptability before you challenge the delusional explanation. This may be a lengthy part of the therapy and may take weeks or even months for patients with no insight.
3. **Always think about what you are doing before you do it** – and do not do it unless you have a good reason for doing it.
4. **Go slowly, be gentle**. Be prepared to back off if necessary. Do not be tempted to press ahead too quickly because you are concerned about lack of apparent progress.

SUPERVISION

Because of the complexity and difficulty of this work, it is strongly recommended that practising therapists join with others for peer supervision.

Clinical psychologists and other qualified CBT therapists make particularly good partners for this type of supervision because their professional training gives them a breadth of background knowledge not only about the principles underlying CBT but also about other models and ways of looking at the patient's presenting problems.

GETTING STARTED

A set of examples has been prepared that take the reader through all the stages of goal setting and treatment for individual patients, explaining what was done in practice, and why. These are available on request from the author.

Appendix 2
Summary of treatment strategies with delusions and hallucinations

COGNITIVE BEHAVIOUR STRATEGIES WITH DELUSIONS

1. **Assessment and setting the goals of therapy.**
2. **Lessening the impact/distress of the delusional ideas.**
3. **Promoting insight:**
    (i)   destigmatising and normalising the symptoms and illness label:
        (a) sharing experiences of 'odd' ideas
        (b) discussing the factors that increase vulnerability to 'odd' ideas
        (c) education about automatic thoughts etc.
        (d) discussing the meaning of 'schizophrenia'
    (ii) experience is not the same as 'fact':
        (a) misinterpretation of everyday events
        (b) beliefs held in the past but no longer held
        (c) misperception at a physiological level, e.g. visual illusions
        (d) use of dream analogy
        (e) imagination is not the same as reality
    (iii) discussion of how and why the delusions might have occurred.
4. **CBT with the non-psychotic beliefs influencing the delusions.**
5. **Modifying (challenging) the delusions:**
    (i)   making the general specific
    (ii) logical reasoning
    (iii) evidence for and against
    (iv) alternative explanations

    (v)   reality testing/experimenting

    (vi) errors/biases in thinking

6. **Long-term strategies:**
   - (i)   encourage recognition and labelling of delusional ideas
   - (ii) develop sets of arguments and challenges to counter specific delusions
   - (iii) develop/enhance coping strategies:
     - (a) develop coping statements
     - (b) develop a set of practical coping behaviours
     - (c) relapse prevention
     - (d) medication compliance
   - (iv) make cards of the above, as appropriate.

COGNITIVE BEHAVIOUR STRATEGIES WITH HALLUCINATIONS

1. **Assessment and setting the goals of therapy.**
2. **Practical ways of reducing the voices:**
   - (i)   personalised cassette player (Walkman)
   - (ii) earplug.
3. **Promoting insight:**
   - (i)   destigmatising and normalising the symptoms and illness label:
     - (a) sharing experiences of voices
     - (b) discussing the factors that increase vulnerability to hearing 'voices'
     - (c) education about automatic thoughts
     - (d) discussing the meaning of 'schizophrenia'
   - (ii) experience is not the same as fact:
     - (a) misinterpretation of everyday events
     - (b) misperception at a physiological level, e.g. visual illusions
     - (c) use of dream analogy
   - (iii) discussion of how and why the voices might have occurred.
4. **CBT with the non-psychotic beliefs influencing the content of the hallucinations.**
5. **Disempowering the voices:**
   - (i)   evidence to disprove what the voices say
   - (ii) voices cannot inflict physical harm
   - (iii) the voices are liars/ignorant
   - (iv) directly question and challenge the voices
   - (v) voices cannot compel action.
6. **Modifying (challenging) the delusional beliefs about the voices:**
   - (i)   making the general specific
   - (ii) logical reasoning

(iii) evidence for and against
(iv) alternative explanations
(v) reality testing/experimenting

7. **Long-term strategies:**
   (i) encourage recognition and labelling of voices
   (ii) develop sets of arguments and challenges to counter the voices
   (iii) develop/enhance coping strategies:
      (a) develop coping statements
      (b) develop a set of practical coping strategies
      (c) relapse prevention
      (d) medication compliance
   (iv) make cards of the above, as appropriate.

Recommended further reading

For comprehensive coverage of the theoretical and research backgrounds to the use of CBT with schizophrenia, as well as discussion of treatment strategies

Chadwick, P.D., Birchwood, M.J. and Trower, P. (1996) *Cognitive Therapy for Delusions, Voices and Paranoia*, Wiley, Chichester.

Fowler, D., Garety, P. and Kuipers, L. (1995) *Cognitive Behaviour Therapy for Psychosis*, Wiley, Chichester.

Haddock, G. and Slade, P.D. (eds) (1996) *Cognitive-Behavioural Interventions with Psychotic Disorders*, Routledge, London.

Kingdon, D.G. and Turkington, D. (1994) *Cognitive-Behavioural Therapy of Schizophrenia*, Lawrence Erlbaum, Hove.

For a recent overview of the use of psychological approaches to schizophrenia

Birchwood, M. and Tarrier, N. (eds) (1994) *Psychological Management of Schizophrenia*, Wiley, Chichester.

For information about the assessment of delusions and hallucinations

Brett-Jones, J., Garety, P. and Hemsley, D. (1987) Measuring delusional experiences: a method and its application. *British Journal of Clinical Psychology*, **26**, 257–65.

Garety, P. and Wessely, S. (1994) The assessment of positive symptoms, in *The Assessment of Psychoses: A Practical Handbook*, (eds T.R.E. Barnes and H.E. Nelson), Chapman & Hall, London, pp. 21–40.

For discussion of medication compliance issues

McPhillips, M.A. and Sensky, T. Coercion, adherence or collaboration? Influences on compliance with medication, in *Outcome and Innovation in Psychological Treatment of Schizophrenia*, (ed. T. Wykes), Wiley, Chichester (in press).

For a recent review of the use of medication with schizophrenia

Hirsch, S.R. and Barnes, T.R.E. (1995) The clinical treatment of schizophrenia with antipsychotic medication, in *Schizophrenia*, (eds S.R. Hirsch and D. Weinberger), Blackwell Scientific Publications, London, pp. 443–68.

For a comprehensive volume of current thinking about the neuropsychology of schizophrenia

Pantelis, C., Nelson, H.E. and Barnes, T.R.E. (eds) (1996) *Schizophrenia: A Neuropsychological Perspective*, Wiley, Chichester.

For information about the role of biosocial systems in human behaviour

Gilbert, P. (1989) *Human Nature and Suffering*, Lawrence Erlbaum, Hove.

For a short but excellent, easy-to-read introduction to the use of CBT with depression

Blackburn, I.M. (1987) *Coping with Depression*, Chambers, Edinburgh.

For a guide to the use of CBT in general clinical practice

Hawton, K., Salkovskis, P.M., Kirk, J. and Clark, D.M. (1989) *Cognitive Behaviour Therapy for Psychiatric Problems: A Practical Guide*, Oxford University Press, Oxford.

Index